Veterinary Management in Transition

Preparing for the Twenty-first Century

OTHER BOOKS BY THOMAS CATANZARO

Building the Successful Veterinary Practice

  Volume 1 • *Leadership Tools*
  Volume 2 • *Programs and Procedures*
  Volume 3 • *Innovation and Creativity*

IOWA STATE UNIVERSITY PRESS / AMES

Veterinary Management in Transition

Preparing for the Twenty-first Century

Thomas E. Catanzaro, DVM, MHA, FACHE
Diplomate, American College of Healthcare Executives

Thomas E. Catanzaro, DVM, MHA, FACHE, Diplomate, American College of Healthcare Executives, received his DVM from Colorado State University and his master's in health care from Baylor University. He is the only veterinarian to have achieved board certification in healthcare administration. Currently president and CEO of Catanzaro & Associates, a veterinary management consulting firm, Catanzaro is in wide demand as consultant and speaker.

© 2000 Iowa State University Press
All rights reserved

Iowa State University Press
2121 South State Avenue, Ames, Iowa 50014

Orders: 1-800-862-6657
Office: 1-515-292-0140
Fax: 1-515-292-3348
Web site: www.isupress.edu

Authorization to photocopy items for internal or personal use, or the internal or personal use of specific clients, is granted by Iowa State University Press, provided that the base fee of $.10 per copy is paid directly to the Copyright Clearance Center, 222 Rosewood Drive, Danvers, MA 01923. For those organizations that have been granted a photocopy license by CCC, a separate system of payments has been arranged. The fee code for users of the Transactional Reporting Service is 0-8138-2626-8/2000 $.10.

♾ Printed on acid-free paper in the United States of America

First edition, 2000

Library of Congress Cataloging-in-Publication Data

Catanzaro, Thomas E.
   Veterinary management in transition: preparing for the twenty-first
century/Thomas E. Catanzaro—1st ed.
      p.   cm.
   ISBN 0-8138-2626-8
   1. Veterinary medicine—Practice.   I. Title.
   SF756.4.C38   1999
   636.089′068—dc21   99-058668

The last digit is the print number: 9 8 7 6 5 4 3 2 1

Contents

CHAPTER FOUR

CHAPTER FIVE

Preface

In early 1998, at the request of some of our Canadian clients, I submitted an article to the *Canadian Veterinary Journal*, entitled, "Beyond the R.K. House Report," and the editor refused to publish the article for being too aggressive. The R.K. House report concluded, from long survey documents submitted to veterinary practitioners and at a great cost to each Province, that veterinarians in Canada were not charging enough for their services. Wonder how they figured that one out?

They started their survey in Manitoba, the equivalent of North Dakota the United States. This means almost all the veterinarians surveyed were mixed animal practitioners, which compounded the fee-for-service problem; we all know that producers deal in cents per hundredweight, but the House report never addressed that issue. To make a long story short, most of our Canadian clients said, "Don't tell us what is wrong, tell us what we can do about it!" So I wrote the article that follows.

Beyond the R.K. House Report

When the only tool you have is a hammer, all problems are approached as if they were nails.
—The Bookkeeper

The landmark R.K. House & Associates practice survey report showed most Canadian practitioners that they were undercharging and explained most of the issues in accounting terms and ratios. There are many ways that money appears in a veterinary hospital, and without it nothing else can occur. In fact without it, the front door gets locked by the bank and it can never swing again. This article is designed to provide the reader a method for reassessing the habits and biases of the years that have gone before. Many perspectives shared herein are from *Building the Successful Veterinary Practice* (text in three volumes, published by Iowa State University Press, 1997–1998) and can be applied to any practice.

The major problem in veterinary medicine is that we are a young profession and are defining the business as we go. The first companion animal hospital was built in 1929, and the American Animal Hospital Association was started in 1938. This means most all practice owners learned from some guy (yes, they were virtually all men way back then) who was in a farm practice and decided to see the smaller companion animals. That is why we call it small animal medicine. Look at the following habits and traditions and the alternatives, and you may start to understand.

- We have routinely scheduled one doctor in one room with a single column of clients, yet physicians use four to six rooms per doctor, and dentists are double that number (now think of the old-time veterinarian, in his truck, doing one farm at a time).

  ✓ The smart practice has started to schedule two consultation rooms concurrently, but out-of-phase, for a doctor-nurse (technician) outpatient team. In four hours, a full day's companion animal workload is possible, thereby allowing time for the equine and producer clients in the normal work day, instead of late into the night.
  ✓ If you believe that we can practice smarter and understand that the staff produces the net while the doctors produce the gross, review High Density Scheduling in Volume 2 of *Building the Successful Veterinary Practice* for some alternative methods.

- We have routinely charged anesthesia by the animal size, yet isoflurane costs only $6 per hour to use (now think of the value of the cow in the chute, the veterinarian and his/her black bag, and the cost per kilogram to make her well).

  ✓ If you want to see the new perspective, consider the following sequence, with each item/procedure deserving its own fair price.

    ✗ Essential pre-anesthetic blood screen (varies with age and physical condition),
    ✗ Induction (less than $20, but covers most overhead),
    ✗ Initial maintenance (not by weight, but for 30 minutes minimum),
    ✗ Continuing anesthesia maintenance (by the minute),
    ✗ Required postsurgery pain medication,
    ✗ Postsurgery hospitalization, and
    ✗ The follow-up plan.

- For some unexplained reason, veterinary medicine made pre-anesthesia blood screening voluntary, made IV supportive therapy during surgery an exception, and always said, "but what about the price?"

  ✓ In quality companion animal practices, the blood screen is now mandatory (thank goodness).
  ✓ In progressive practices that worry about animal pain and rapid recovery, supportive IV therapy [IV TKO (to keep open)] during surgery is mandatory.
  ✓ The full, traditional, pricing is secondary to the needs of the patient and the provider in terms of quality—compromise of professional standards is a liability. A surgical IV is a butterfly and a slow drip of about 100 ml of fluid—a very inexpensive cost to the practice and even to the client at 2.5 times markup.

- We have always charged hospitalization cage and run space by the animal size (almost like a feedlot operation).

  ✓ The value is in the time, process, and people involved, not the kibble in the bowl:

    ✗ o.d./b.i.d. cases—level one hospitalization
    ✗ t.i.d./q.i.d.—level two hospitalization
    ✗ IV—level three hospitalization (also postsurgery)
    ✗ ICU—level four hospitalization

  ✓ Yes, this can be used in bandaging (no joint, one joint, two joints, with an appliance or supportive wrap or without)—start rethinking your habits.

- We have always been afraid to sell our knowledge and, instead, have routinely sold things (e.g., vaccines at major inflation markups, the cost of the exam instead of the doctor's consultation, etc.).

  ✓ Producer veterinarians have started charging for their time, even on the telephone, with clients.
  ✓ Producer veterinarians have started software computer systems to manage the husbandry for their clients, and they charge for this service.
  ✓ Producer and farm veterinarians charge by the mile to get to a client, yet house-call veterinarians and mobile specialists who travel between companion animal practices usually have not.
  ✓ When the pendulum starts to swing, why do the companion

animal veterinarians always wait for the other guys to change first?

- We have always managed companion animal practices by expense comparisons, yet the traditional veterinary software has been like a very fancy cash register, only tracking income factors (and providing a mail merge feature for client mailings).

  - ✓ Without expense to income relationships, you cannot determine net.
  - ✓ Program-based budgeting provides program and procedure factors for managing practices—the things that make the front door swing.
  - ✓ The new veterinary software systems, in 32-bit Windows technology, will track healthcare delivery, in picture and word, and the better systems will also have automatic data download capabilities to existing spreadsheet programs for easy practice use.

Now let's look at one simple continuity-of-care example, with fees, and see where your practice has positioned itself. First, every animal that comes into the companion animal practice deserves to be weighed, receive a nurse's wellness screen, and have the teeth graded. We recommend using the four pictures and descriptions on the back of a common vendor dental handout brochure for grading, so the client can take the picture home to the family for further discussion. Second, the staff explains the grades in terms of pain and bad breath, not periodontal disease and gingivitis (doctor talk that confuses most clients). Third, the doctor endorses the nurse technician as the dental hygiene counselor, thereby releasing him/herself to the next case and allowing the staff to continue the care and client education process. So how does this work in a real practice setting? Here is an example.

- We have always charged one rate for dental procedures, but look at what our staff must do in each case when we grade teeth (it is not like floating teeth in horses).

  - ✓ The value is in the time, process, and people involved (the dollar values are only starting examples, and grade two must be set on the community standard since dental care is becoming a commodity (quotable) item):

    - ✗ $85 *Grade 1+* —white teeth, red gums, a little molar color; a condition usually medically ignored, although red indicates pain. This is the beginning of bad breath, and the client **must** be told!

✗ $135   *Grade 2+*—(where you are probably currently setting your fees) brown teeth. Bad breath and pain are very evident, tell the client!

✗ $195   *Grade 3+*—tartar buildup, real bad breath, a lot of pain, extractions expected, and a very hard mouth to clean. Radiographs are needed and will be an additional fee.

✗ >$300   *Grade 4+*—all of the above and down into the bone, with major infection and systemic concerns. This will require a major correction and a protracted medical care program.

✓ If this system is used, and if the dental grade is recorded in the medical record every time, the number of dental procedures will increase, the quality of health care will be enhanced, and most importantly, the other people in the practice will know what was said previously and will start from that point when talking with the client.

So yes, more money does matter, but it comes from quality health-care delivery and new perspectives, not just from charging a higher fee for the same things. Liquidity must be captured from the work we do. It is not just the average client transaction (ACT) or revenue per visit (RPV); rather, it is the number of visits per year per client. It is setting the expectation for the next contact or scheduling the next visit, not just selling some extra pet food or shampoo. Veterinary medicine is a fee-for-service business: products are only supportive. And in companion animal practice, we generally treat patients that are considered family members (as shown in the original family value research published in *The Pet Connection*, CENSHARE, University of Minnesota, and more recently in the Pfizer survey of 38,000-plus veterinary clients). We deal in needs, those of the patient, the client, and the provider. The 1997 Pfizer study also showed that over 85 percent of the clients wanted a 20-minute **or less** consultation room episode. That means that violating the social contract of an appointment is not only inappropriate, it is dangerous, especially when there is another practice that keeps its word to busy clients.

So as you look at the accountant's figures, please remember that he/she has never palpated a cow, never stood at the exam table, never counseled a client in grief. The accountant knows where you wrote the checks and for how much. He/she doesn't know how to schedule the return visit, how to ask about other companion animals at home, or how to pass a case to a staff member for sequential monthly weights, parasite prevention and control counseling, or dental hygiene follow-up. Accountants deal in expenses, so the financial reports seldom match income centers to expense centers, thereby hiding net income evaluations from the practice. Veterinary practice is a business which requires timely reports of the cost of delivering a specific service, which then allows rationale decisions about what fees to charge. Quit using a hammer to make the fees increase. Become innovative and creative in your quest for healthcare excellence. Start using the professional knowledge at your finger tips and in your heart, train the staff to be trusted, thereby extending your healthcare effect, and challenge the old habits that have gotten you where you are today.

And the above Article Was Too Radical for Canada!

I tell you this story to put this book into perspective. Most everything in the above article was from the Iowa State University Press series *Building the Successful Veterinary Practice*. We are well aware that not everyone will agree with me, or even with what I predict for management transitions. That is okay; in fact, I would worry if everyone agreed with me. Our consulting firm has chosen to take the high road in this profession and in veterinary practice consulting. Leadership will be the linchpin for success in the next millennium. Leveraging the staff as veterinary extenders will be a major net income source. Focusing on client and community needs, rather than practice stability and traditional habits, will be the key to retaining the practice's most valuable assets, the staff members.

I have achieved a fellowship status within the American College of Healthcare Executives (only about 10 percent of the 30,000-plus members have achieved this recognition in ACHE) and have maintained my diplomate status in ACHE because they have already done what we are trying to do. Board certification at ACHE must be renewed every five years, and by taking the oral and written ACHE boards, in the 10 major areas of healthcare administration interest (see Appendix B), I must verify to the governing body and myself that I am staying current. I have nominated many of my veterinary medical consulting colleagues as candidates for these ACHE boards, but to date none have accepted the challenge. A few have accepted the Certified Veterinary Practice

Manager (CVPM) challenge, for the oral and written boards offered by the Veterinary Hospital Managers Association board, and I consider that a significant accomplishment, which is laudatory and very appropriate for anyone who holds him/herself out as a consultant in this profession.

Regardless of their credentials, this book is dedicated to those managers and administrators of tomorrow who will enter the new millennium as educators of the curmudgeons and traditionalists. It is dedicated to the consulting leaders of our profession, such as the associates of Veterinary Practice Consultants (web address: <www.v-p-c.com>). It is dedicated to those practice leaders in our caring and compassionate profession, those who will help turn veterinary practices into small business operations. It is dedicated to those veterinary practices which are evolving into contemporary business operations, organizations which can generate adequate funds to remunerate the staff, doctors, and business owners, as well as support the community and patients, in an appropriate manner, while never losing the caring and compassion of patient advocates.

Author's Note: If you are reading this text and have not read *Building the Successful Veterinary Practice,* a three-volume, leadership-based, practice management series released by ISU Press in 1997–1998, some application assumptions made by the reader may prove very confusing and misleading.

INTRODUCTION

Are You an Effective Veterinary Administrator?

The Veterinary Healthcare Team

Leadership is action, not position.
—Dr. T.E. Catanzaro

The position titles of technician, receptionist, technician assistant, kennel staff, animal caretaker, pet love specialist, practice manager, hospital manager, business manager, office manager, hospital administrator, and contract practice manager mean different things to different people. Let's try to get some idea of what we mean by starting with some Veterinary Hospital Managers Association (VHMA @ 518-433-8911) definitions, augmented by Veterinary Practice Consultants® to meet more of the variations observed in the "real" practice world:

- *Hospital administrator.* Not defined originally by VHMA, but defined by this author as a person with complete authority over the business and operations of the practice under direction of the owners/board; final authority in fiscal decisions; supervision of all practice activities. Coordinating agent for facility use and expansion planning; medical protocols short of therapeutic decisions; continuity of care; and all functions of other managers and administrators listed below.

- *Practice manager.* Person who possesses all the knowledge of an office manager plus has direct authority and decision-making responsibilities over all business activities and practice internal promotions.

- *Contract practice manager.* A management person outside the staff structure but on contract to the practice; manages multiple practices within a geographic region, with the proven knowledge and skills of a practice manager or higher [e.g., Certified Veterinary Practice Manager (CVPM) designation awarded by the VHMA].

- *Hospital manager.* Not defined by VHMA, but generally similar to a practice manager.

- *Office manager.* Person who handles daily accounting, banking, schedule coordination, purchasing, training, directing the front office staff, and client relations.

- *Business manager.* Not defined by VHMA, but similar to an office manager with a heavier bookkeeping and budget-monitoring role and fewer staff supervision functions.

- *Administrative assistant.* Designation generally reserved for a staff person who works within a single practice but is trained and directed by an outside contract management person; jointly supervised by contract practice manager and facility owner/director(s).

The above definitions aside, there are multiple other practice management categories; some say there are as many as the creative mind can imagine. When coordination is needed, somebody will get the nod, and maybe a title. These workers are called program managers in the rest of the world; in the new millennium veterinary practice, these paraprofessionals are often called the *management team* and may in the future be called the *leadership team.* Management or leadership teams may include any of the following:

- *Program manager.* This leadership team member is accountable for the improvement of the results of a specific practice program (e.g., inventory, reminders, nutritional counseling, etc.). In the average practice (2.6 doctors, less than a million dollars gross, with about 1,000 transactions a month), the program manager usually has additional duties, such as those listed below.

- *Technician (nurse).* This person can be licensed, registered, certified (term is state or province specific), and they could have been on-the-job or school trained, another variable within the State or Province sanction system. Currently, the American Veterinary Medical Association segregates these paraprofessionals by education (technologist, four years; technician, two years; and assistant, trained on the job), but clients understand the term *nurse.* These are skilled professionals who can support the delivery of veterinary health care and also monitor the regulatory medicine requirements of the DEA, FDA, EPA, ADA, and OSHA or WHIMS. The bottom line is that they are concerned with quality patient care and facility safety, and they extend the healthcare delivery capabilities of the doctor(s) in accordance with the practice philosophy.

- *Technical assistant.* Someone without all the skills needed to operate independently, but who is assigned to help others work with patients in the treatment room or consultation room.

- *Receptionist (secretary).* Some practices call these special people client relations specialists; the name should add pride, not frustration. This staff member should be a caring, people person, a smiling face who greets clients, handles the phone, and coordinates the front desk activities. Computer literacy is becoming a must.

- *Animal caretaker.* This is the pooper scooper, the bather, the comb-out specialist, and the person who helps maintain the facility and the grounds. This person may be a technician assistant in practices with only a few cages. Animal caretakers should be the experts in compliance to Title 9, CFR, Subchapter A (the Animal Welfare Act).

- *Pet love specialist.* A cute name for an adoption specialist, this person is someone who understands pet placement, the liability of adoption activities, and family or individual needs for the human/animal bond. He or she may also be a technician, or a receptionist, or even another skilled paraprofessional on the team.

Office Manager, Practice Manager, or Hospital Administrator; the difference lies in the commitment, not the job description!
—Dr. T.E. Catanzaro

To summarize, the veterinary healthcare team is everyone inside the practice's operational structure; some of these individuals become managers, some administrators, and some leaders. The job title is not as important as trust in the individual, and responsibility is not as important as accountability. Although responsibility, shared by the practice owner(s) and the leadership team, is important, it is accountability for outcomes that is the cornerstone of an effective team. As part of this system, compensation for any individual is **always** negotiable; real leaders may ask for and receive a portion of the excess savings and/or excess earnings of the practice, but they do not ask for guarantees up front. Despite emerging changes in leadership philosophy, delineation of responsibility, accountability, and compensation remains within the practice owner's control; the philosophy shared below is simply the emerging philosophy of leadership for the next millennium. The job description in progressive practices for managers/administrators could simply read, "Identify/solve/prevent problems; see the need for and make continual quality improvements." This is the road to leadership.

When you are trying to find a good horse, you have to
go to a lot of sales and trade often. When you get the right
one, you stop shopping and pour your effort into developing
that one as your partner.
—Joe Green

The New Era

The days of successful one-doctor practices are coming to an end. It will not fit with either the economies of scale or the demand for a balanced life seen with new associates and staff members. No single-doctor practice can keep the doors open and the clients supported without sacrificing some quality of life or quality patient health care. This is not a great decision to ask of any healthcare professional or staff member. Remember,

Families are forever; practice is short-term!
—Dr. T.E. Catanzaro

Furthermore, practices are becoming more client centered, and our national associations are publishing staff support aids which support this observation. If the client-centered service is being driven to the staff level, so must the leadership of the practice. The single-doctor habit of total practice control must be relinquished when the practice expands beyond the single-doctor format. The quality-of-life sacrifice, tenacity, and vision of one doctor that it takes to make a start-up practice successful will often prevent the success of a multi-doctor practice (where sharing leadership, compromise, and ensuring quality of life for all are essential).

As a veterinary healthcare administrator, are you concerned about your career success? Do you look forward to expanding your daily responsibilities, to moving to a larger veterinary facility that will let you expand your capabilities? Are you an individual who is interested in increasing your own effectiveness right where you are so you can survive another year? If so, there is probably nothing more interesting to you than increasing your own capabilities and enhancing your administrative effectiveness. Therefore, we need to explore the following questions: What is effectiveness for a veterinary healthcare professional? What is the role of the veterinary administrator in the new millennium? Where are the management expectations evolving?

The Prime Thrust: Effective Administration

In healthcare, effectiveness resides in the ability to direct the veterinary practice resources by pinpointing the efforts of the paraprofessional team toward opportunities for significant results. In an administrator's development, this increases personal leverage, allows the expansion of responsibilities and accountabilities, and makes the practice an effective veterinary healthcare delivery system in his/her community.

An effective administrator primarily focuses on opportunities rather than problems. (Crisis management never moved a veterinary practice forward.) Secondly, he/she puts effort into areas that have maximum impact on the effectiveness of the practice. Time is not misallocated to process management; it is used to make the front door swing, increase staff pride, or do quality assurance spot checks on cost-benefit assessment of income centers. In veterinary practices across the United States, there has been a fundamental confusion between efficiency and effectiveness. A good veterinary healthcare administrator wants to be effective, not just efficient.

To paraphrase Peter Drucker, the efficient veterinary practice manager focuses on doing things right for the veterinarian, but the effective administrator focuses on doing the right things for the practice. Doing the right things puts the focus on what can increase the perception of wellness, caring, and service while increasing the return on investment (time, staff and/or money). There is no need to hang onto sclerotic procedures, habits, or practices because "this is the way we have always done it around this practice." Instead, an effective healthcare administrator is concerned with wellness outcomes (satisfied clients, proud staff, and net income), continuous quality improvement (CQI) by the staff, and individuals *being* good rather than just *looking* good. He/she is more interested in helping individuals achieve results that help the practice than in simply keeping people busy. Such administrators understand that internal processes must be fluid enough to promote client returns. As a result, changes are made based on outcome evaluations, not on input requirements.

Signs of Administrative Success and Failure

Earmarks of the Downward Spiral

There are many practice-specific indicators of a failing veterinary hospital administrator. Although these indicators vary by practice and practice owner, there are also a few universal signs:

- *High turnover of staff*. If the veterinary practice is within 10 percent of the community average for turnover, the practice is in trouble. Veterinary practices should have turnover rates far below the community average because of their commitment to a caring profession.

- *A reactor profile*. Someone who lets events, crises, and constant problems dissipate his/her time is a reactor. Sometimes a reactor is concurrently an actor, and the action is masked. If you suspect someone is a reactor, evaluate the level of planning he/she does. Specifically, determine whether the suspected reactor establishes preventive procedures that routinize events, thus allowing other people to handle problem issues in due course. Reactors do not plan objectives, set standards of performance ahead of time, or know what good work is until they see it. They clearly communicate neither practice needs nor personal expectations.

- *Demand for conformity*. Failing administrators need emotional support for their authority. As a result, control of the environment, rather than getting a good return on the human assets invested, becomes a primary goal of the panicked manager. A "manager" delegates specific task processes instead of clearly defining the expected outcomes and letting the team members doing the job decide the process. Managers see open communication, where disagreement as well as agreement can be expressed, as disturbing or counterproductive, not as using the resources of the group. A manager shares blame by assigning it to someone else rather than accepting accountability for misadventures and nurturing the team.

- *Lack of mistakes*. One of the strongest signs of a failing veterinary practice administrator is that he/she maintains the status quo.

Insistence (often by the veterinarian) on maintaining the status quo decreases initiative and avoids risk and confrontation. In this situation, the "manager" makes all the decisions and does not want new ideas. Since no one is willing to risk telling the manager anything, the staff waits for signals and signs from the manager before taking safe action. This problem is often manifested by people being really good at whatever they are told to do but never volunteering or taking initiative to make improvements.

- *Getting by.* The traditional habit of surviving a day at a time will not work in the new millennium. Raising quality and operational standards, on an incremental and continuous basis, will be the foundation of success. The status-quo quest of twentieth century veterinary management will likely be the death knell of many practices. The profession is adding diagnostic tools and medical knowledge on applications of screening procedures at an alarming rate (alarming because the continuing education requirements are now required of most every provider to just stay even in the profession). Continuous quality improvement (CQI) must become the hospital administrator's primary tool for practice transition.

Signs of a Winner

Successful administrators are those who exceed the expectations of the veterinarian/owner. The earmarks of a successful administrator, like those of a failing administrator, are highly variable, but winners do have some common traits:

- *Accountability.* Here, accountability is not defined as accepting responsibility and authority for delegated tasks. Accountability is an atmosphere created by a skillful veterinary practice administrator who looks beyond task and process. This winning administrator assigns outcome-oriented accountabilities that allow every team member to take ownership of some element of practice success. This continuous quality improvement (CQI) concept allows pride to become the individual's input while the client's perception of quality becomes the output.

- *Commitment.* A winner commits to excellence, and performance competency is equated with doing the best job possible. Performance appraisals are based on a single standard of performance established for the task, not the individual. The veterinary practice's administrator accepts the commitment to ensure that each team member has the opportunity to train to a level of competency that sets the standard for the profession.

- *Time management.* The effective veterinary facility administrator allocates time by investing it rather than spending it. Such an administrator accepts the fact that time does not stretch or shrink and sees time management as simply scheduling events in a more effective manner. Overtime is well controlled and space is utilized by plan, not by tradition or chance. When time becomes dissipated by process, poor planning, inadequate space utilization, or crisis management, the performance of both the administrator and the staff suffers. The skilled administrator understands that one hour of planning saves at least four hours of mistakes and corrections.

- *Guts to cut.* A competent and confident veterinary practice administrator has the courage to amputate those activities, non-contributing projects, and processes that dissipate time, waste resources, or frustrate clients. The role of the administrative surgeon is to remove these debilitating practice appendages early, before they can harm the practice. To change the undesirable habits of either the veterinarian or the staff, the effective veterinary practice administrator will use a calculated and caring process of sharing information, negotiating slowly to form a discomfort with the undesirable habit, then offering alternative solutions to the habit-based problem.

- *Empowering, not directing.* The traditional veterinary hospital manager of the twentieth century built so many job descriptions and procedure manuals that the staff member never had to think. This practice came from the World War II training standards. Although all training starts out very directive, leaders follow the directive stage with persuasive sessions that convince the staff member that he/she can do the job. Then the leader moves into a coaching mode, giving guidance on how to better achieve desired outcomes. Setting the outcome expectations in a clearly defined, time-line based, joint-discussion manner is the key to delegation of authority and empowerment. Using the outcome orientation rather than a defined process, with a joint agreement on success measures **before** the project or program starts, results in staff empowerment, continuous improvement, and a success that will be shared and celebrated throughout the practice.

Applying Effectiveness Concepts

A modern healthcare administrator promotes quality healthcare delivery while ensuring adequate remuneration for the facility and establishing a clear market niche in the community. To the administrator, this means letting people do more than the job they were hired for. If the people on the payroll are to be the ones to make things happen, they must become the problem solvers. A good healthcare administrator just keeps the impeding habits out of the way. A great administrator makes change and innovation the expectation for each staff member.

Self-evaluation

The basic operational questions which effective veterinary practice administrators ask themselves each day include the following:

- Today, what projects and objectives need to be accomplished and what needs must be met in this facility?

- Have we established staff members as the primary users of our emerging programs and procedures, rather than as expendable employees? What have we done today to make them feel significant?

- What will I facilitate by removing obstacles from the path of our team?

- How can I further my transition from the person with the great answers to all problems to an administrator who asks great questions of staff members that empower their solution-finding capabilities? What are the good questions I need to ask today?

- Since I am the steward of administrative talents for this practice, which staff members need my help to develop their skills and success rates further today?

- What is the practice standard that is being established? Do we want a team of people who don't stumble when they walk through their daily duties, or do we want to develop a team of runners who are marathon quality when attacking problems?

- When staff members walk through my door with a problem on their back, have I developed the mental position to be reactive or proactive? How can I ensure they leave with both the problem and some alternatives still on their back, with accountability for resolution in their hands?

Appreciating Human Resources

Human resources are the only practice asset that can be appreciated rather than depreciated, and the savvy administrator treats these human resources, both clients and staff, as valuable assets. The effective veterinary practice administrator becomes a significant other to each team member. He/she is a sounding board who helps staff members think through the problems and discover alternatives. The best administrator validates the thought process often enough that every staff member learns not only to solve problems and make the practice better without asking permission, but also to act before problems occur. They make their environment more user (staff and client) friendly on a daily basis. In other words, their value appreciates.

In applying leadership skills within the practice's healthcare delivery team, the effective veterinary practice administrator follows the three Bs, offering staff the chance "to be, to belong, and to become." Team members are given a chance *to be* a recognized somebody rather than a nobody who is taken for granted. They are given a chance *to belong*, to be part of the practice success system rather than just a pair of hands. Finally, they are given a chance *to become* capable of doing greater things as an individual and as a member of the practice team, to be able to stretch their necks out without fear of injury. A person who has captured and embraced all three Bs, as they were provided by the administrator, may develop as a replacement or backup to that administrator. Such employees have had their well-being nurtured, and they know they can enrich themselves and their lives through work and practice progress rather than just through off-the-job educational opportunities.

We all need to remember that staff members were hired because someone in the practice liked their skills and attitude. A staff member with a bad attitude is one who has been depreciated by the practice rather than appreciated. The veterinary administrator is a people person who can cause human resources to appreciate by focusing on outcomes rather than process and by sharing control of the practice with the staff.

The Future

The Role of Hospital Managers in Veterinary Medicine

Veterinary medicine is an art, and art doesn't need managers, it needs artists. Veterinary practice is an art and a science, and it has some facets that need to be managed. In most cases, a veterinary facility is a small business operation that requires competent management to ensure some form of profitability and longevity. Facility administrators must realize that veterinary healthcare delivery is one of the service industries in America and must respond to the market demands. Successful practices today aren't just high quality practices; they are practices that communicate high quality to clients, and that make management of the information systems available to the practice.

In the interest of effective management, certain texts should be required reading for veterinary administrators who wish to build and/or maintain successful hospital practices. *Service America,* by Albrect and Zemke, needs to be on every hospital director's reading list. It needs to be read at least annually and applied to the business of veterinary healthcare delivery. In addition, *The Veterinary Hospital Manual,* provided by Kal Kan Foods, Inc., for less than $10, should be in every technician's library. *Building the Successful Veterinary Practice: Innovation and Creativity*, from ISU Press, may also be useful for veterinary hospital managers who want to become veterinary hospital administrators of larger organizations.

Revolutionary Change

The evolution of veterinary practices is over—we are now in a revolution. The slow progressive changes made famous by Darwin and his finches cannot be seen in veterinary practice today; the environment is changing too fast. The practice must be ready to manage its own future. The revolution of change requires that time management become a factor of daily professional practice efficiency. The hospital director is worth greater than $2.00 per minute when providing patient care in the exam room or surgery; even the best paid manager is worth only $0.20 per minute for the toughest of the administrative challenges handled in a practice. Take a look at where the veterinarians in your practice are spending their time and compute what they are worth to the practice. Sit down and review realistically who manages that new nutritional center; who provides the behavior counseling services; who does the dental hygiene training; who does bank deposits, scheduling, and maintenance; and even, who does animal exercise and cleansing duties.

Dealing with Management Costs

The future is based on today, for if we don't learn from history we will be sure to repeat it. Some consultants recommend an average of 10 percent of the gross be set aside as a management expense factor; other astute CPA consultants show that managerial salaries average only about 3.5 percent of the gross. The future will probably prove the latter figure to be more true, although examination of the owner's draw will reveal a portion that will make the first figure seem more appropriate for budgeting purposes.

Since we are discussing the specific future of veterinary hospital managers, look to the math. Can 3.5 percent of the practice gross support a competent individual and his/her family? If not, could partial management fees be added to existing key staff members' salaries to ensure that specific portions of the management needs have managers that care about efficient completion of the assigned tasks? Be creative, it will cause excitement within the staff.

The national average last year, in the current publications, reflected that about 35 percent of the practices had dedicated managers, most being paid in the $22,000–29,000 range. Salaries of true administrators were in the $45,000–55,000 range, before performance incentives (or bonus monies) were added. Salaries in Alaska and California were higher, but what else would you expect?

Impediments to Success

The success of a veterinary practice manager is limited by how willing the hospital director is to let go of control. In many practices, the transfer of control is initiated as an incremental process and carried out at almost a Darwinian pace. This procedure is usually detrimental, and these practices are frequently the same ones that report no significant changes when a hospital manager is added to the staff.

The source of the manager can also be an impediment to success. In most cases, the spouse of the hospital director is less than effective as a team builder. In fact, spouse managers often fit the famous adage, "Managers are those that take credit and give blame, while leaders are those that give credit and take blame." On the other hand, when we take a great technician or a caring receptionist and make him/her our hospital manager, that person may fail because he/she is above his/her level of competence (or comfort). Finally, those managers we hire from the outside world may forget that veterinary health care includes a covenant of caring that makes our clients far more special, and susceptible, than mere customers.

On the flip side of the story, spouses, technicians, receptionists, and outside business college graduates have also made great hospital managers. The unique ability of every veterinary practice team to be different makes success or failure a very personal experience, specific in its details to the practice in question; this is compounded by variability in practice philosophies, scope of services, and comfort zones for the delegation of authority.

THE HOSPITAL MANAGER'S FUTURE QUIZ

As you read the survey, mark the factors that now exist in your specific practice. To ensure that you are being candid and truthful, make copies of it and share them with your staff. Take credit for only those items that have 90 percent concurrence by the staff members. The interpretations of the test responses are on the following page (don't peek please).

____ Staff members readily contribute from their experience and listen to the contributions of others.

____ Conflicts arising from different points of view are considered helpful and are resolved constructively by the staff.

____ Staff members challenge suggestions they believe are unsupported by fact or logic, but avoid arguing just to have their way.

____ Poor solutions are not supported just for the sake of staff harmony or agreement.

____ Differences of staff opinion are discussed and resolved. Coin tossing, averaging, majority vote, and similar cop-outs are avoided when making a decision.

____ Every staff member strives to make the problem-solving process efficient and is careful to facilitate rather than hinder discussion.

____ Staff members encourage and support coworkers who may be reluctant to offer ideas.

____ Staff members understand the value of time and work at eliminating extraneous and/or repetitious discussion.

____ Staff decisions are not arbitrarily overruled by the leader simply because he/she does not agree with them.

____ The staff understands the hospital director will make the best decision he/she can, if a satisfactory staff solution is not forthcoming.

SCORING

1. Count the number of marks in the series of statements on the quiz.

- If the total number marked is less than five, a qualified hospital manager is not likely to be successful in the current environment.

- If there are five to seven items marked, the experienced hospital manager will likely survive and take some of the burden off the hospital director's shoulders.

- If you marked more than seven items, a dedicated hospital administrator will likely be a greatly appreciated asset to the practice and will be able to contribute to the future success of the hospital programs.

2. Discuss the reasons for the densities or lack of densities of staff opinion. Administer the quiz again in 90 days to determine trend changes.

Veterinary Management in Transition

Preparing for the Twenty-first Century

1

Are You Ready to Change?

Nothing happens without transformation!
—W. Ed Deming

It Is Not, Nor Will It Ever Be Again, "Business as Usual"

When I first thought about this text about two years ago, it seemed an easy task to write about what was happening in the veterinary profession. All I needed to do was develop a vision of what this profession would be in the next millennium and write about how to manage veterinary healthcare delivery in that environment. I have, however, been amazed at the changes taking place in veterinary health care in just the past 12 months, and these rapid changes have caused me to reexamine, in this presentation, the major premises of veterinary practice management.

In architecture, form follows function, but in practice, structure follows strategy, and veterinary practice strategies have been changing. Within the equine practice sector, I found a referral hospital diversity that appeared to be a unique spectrum within a single segment of this profession. These hospitals followed neither the companion animal specialty hospital model nor the human healthcare model, since specific trainers can access the hospital multiple times with the same need, due to large brood mare farms, expanded racing strings, and the consolidation of the industry. Furthermore, in the racing and breeding circuits, horse owners are often **never** known to the veterinarians.

There are also new specialty hospitals in which companion animal specialists are affiliated in the same facility for economies of scale. These specialists have, however, often confused the real estate investment with a guarantee of square foot floor space in a hospital. The act of investing in land and building means putting hard capital into a build-to-suit, or as seen with *Field of Dreams,* a build-it-and-they-shall-come venture. The act of affiliation requires harmony and a governance board that wields the sword of Solomon when the specialists try to protect their turf and infringe on others. These specialty hospi-

3

tals are at least as diversified as the equine referral hospitals, and more so in most cases due to the wide variety of community and specialist mixes that are emerging.

As we conduct seminars and consult in practices (now well over 1,200 companion animal, mixed animal, production animal, and equine practices in the past decade), we find that we must change cynicism to optimism before we can effect real changes in a practice. Although frustration is always felt, habits are so ingrained that a resolution cannot be seen. In addition, fear of failure prevents the transition to new management styles in most practices, so the consulting team must assume the mantle of transition guidance experts. In the cases of both equine and companion animal specialty hospitals, problems are emerging every day, turf wars are always lurking, and procedures manuals are not that specific. Most veterinary practice managers have not been prepared to be as diversified as they need to be in this new situation, nor have they been empowered to unilaterally impose a resolution. The new millennium's veterinary administrators will not only have the required skills and knowledge for functioning in this diversified environment. They will also have a win-win attitude and be empowered to "make it happen." We have developed this text reference so veterinary managers will not feel alone, and so they can evolve into effective hospital administrators rather than directed crank turners in a go-nowhere practice setting.

As we enter this new arena of diversity and ever-demanding change, a few basic questions must be answered for each practice team:

- Who is the target client?

- What are the key services and products?

- In which market will you operate?

- What are your specific strategies for differentiation?

- Which are the new directions that must be addressed?

- What is the economic share value of each decision?

Since we live in a time of sound bites, here are a few facts to remember:

- Leadership means managing change; management means mentoring operational diversity.

- The L in quality stands for leadership; clients cannot effectively evaluate quality, but they can easily see staff pride. Staff pride becomes the key quality factor that sways the client's opinion of value for services/products rendered. The staff members are a veterinary practice's most important clients!

- Effective communication means *getting* as well as *giving* information, and most communication is non-verbal, often causing mixed messages to be shared, especially in stressful situations.

- Staff meetings have published agendas, are held at least monthly, and are led by staff members, not owners! Regular meetings allow (and in fact require) staff members to solve the "problem of the month" during the last half of the meeting, and then take ownership of the outcome resolution.

- The uncommon leader uses practice changes to develop people through the work effort. He/she **never** just gets work done through people.

- The strategic response to a passing opportunity should be a *get to* rather than a *got to*—a positive rather than a negative mind set.

- A 5 percent increase in staff morale yields a 2 percent increase in client satisfaction, which causes a 0.5 percent increase in profits.

- Birthday celebrations are important, and a letter acknowledging the event and giving the staff member personal recognition gives the leader a once-a-year chance to be innovative and targeted in setting an example with each staff member.

- Operational excellence is no longer just a differentiation, it is a benchmark mediated by the World Wide Web. There is no option to this criteria!

- Quality care means being a client-centered patient advocate. Only trained veterinary practice professionals can speak for what the patient needs, and they must be very clear about needs when talking to the client. Words and phrases that cloud the issues and confuse the client (such as *recommend, it would be best that,* and *you should consider)* must be replaced by a need statement followed by silence. Listening to the client before, during, and after each healthcare issue allows better healthcare selections (thus more profit).

- Vacation and sick days have died a timely death. Sick days made people have to "get sick" unexpectedly to get what they earned.

Now we group them all together as personal days, award 1 hour for every 20 scheduled hours worked, and let everyone (part-time or full-time) accumulate time for their own scheduled rest and recuperation, and if they get sick, it comes from the same pot of accrued personal days.

- Intellectual capital resides within every staff member. If it is wasted, the return on investment is never captured. An uncommon leader must utilize every neuron in the environment and cause synergy to capture the best return on the investment.

- Part-time hire is giving way to job share positions, where, in the old nomenclature, two part-time people share the accountability between themselves to ensure the job(s) gets done in an appropriate and timely manner. This is why they accumulate the personal days and other training benefits, although at a reduced rate: they are accountable for outcome successes.

- Internally grown veterinary practice managers are being replaced by Certified Veterinary Practice Managers (adequately prequalified candidates who have gone through a peer review examination process sponsored by the Veterinary Hospital Managers Association). And in some large, multidisciplinary facilities, hospital administrators are emerging as the new breed (e.g., Master in Healthcare Administration, board certified by the American College of Healthcare Executives by oral and written examination, required to be renewed every five years). The tradition of staff promotion, usually on the basis of tenure, to a higher level of stress (and often a new level of incompetence) is being replaced. Choice of managers and administrators on the basis of a proven set of administrative and leadership talents that have been tested and verified by a certifying body (e.g., only VHMA and ACHE at the time of this writing) is replacing the staff promotion tradition.

Five Success Measures

When we do a consultation, people always ask for the yardstick of success. They want to know how their practice measures up the experience of the consultant. The standard answer is, "It is an internal measurement, and it depends strictly on your personal goals and objectives, the accomplishment rate of those goals and objectives, and the degree of 'buy-in' from the staff so it will continue without the leader's direct interaction on a moment-by-moment basis." This answer is frustrating, since most practice leaders have not developed a program-based budget, do not have practice-wide shared expectations, and have not even developed an in-service training program to develop the intellectual capital of the team. So for the sake of this text, there can be five major goal areas identified that are generic success measures:

- Profitability

- Return on investment (ROI)

- Productivity (net revenue per FTE staff and/or FTE doctor)

- Innovation (percent of earnings from new services/products)

- Social goals

We are living in fascinating times. Opportunities are abundant, if we let go of the tree trunk and explore the new territory at the end of the limbs. Most traditional veterinarians will not only keep holding the tree trunk, they will throw an ax at anyone who lets go and tries to explore on their own. But there are always those few who make the foray into the unknown, prove it is safe, and blaze the trail for others to follow. In the American business environment, a recent *Wall Street Journal* article stated, "Everybody's under pressure. Some are being healthy, they are exercising and running. Some are building learning organizations and making others successful. Some people are just eating more chocolate." In other words, for some it is the best of times, while for others it is the worst of times.

The veterinary profession is no different—it is dependent on mindset and on the core value application process. For those eating chocolate, it seems the endless practice repositioning, compelled by an ever-changing community, has produced an instability and loss of control that is adversely affecting their lives and their futures. Mere survival has become their highest hope. While this reaction is understandable, and probably warranted in practices where the me-too form of management change is practiced, there are practices that are thriving. Under the same sets of conditions and community influences, there are veterinary practices growing and prospering. Let's set two scenarios:

Practice One: The owner overbuilt a new facility without an operational plan. After the debt was overwhelming, the owner called us for immediate consulting assistance. We tailored a transition plan and laid out the steps to success, as jointly defined by the practice owner and the consulting team. The practice owner stated he had no money for the accounts payable, but meanwhile continued taking a European vacation, ski holidays, and frequent out-of-state continuing education trips (at least quarterly), none of which ever changed his practice style. After the owner reviewed the plan, he immediately made excuses about why he could not change the interior influences, and he called the community needs insignificant (so he didn't have to personally change); then he arbitrarily cherry picked ideas from the plan without any staff involvement or training. As a result, the staff turnover was almost total every six months, and the practice's financial success was only a 20 percent growth.

Practice Two: This practice is an affiliation of five practices into a new common facility, but they started with a call to us to guide the endeavor. The investment group was immediately separated from the hospital operational planning group (governance board). Core values were discussed, defined, and established in writing before debates occurred; clear core values make hard decisions easier. The needs assessment for space in the new facility included a consultant-mediated joint-use and common-use discussion. Equipment limited liability corporation (LLC) entities were established so fair market values (FMV) were established, and leases were written defining the new business relationships. Planning allowed a cost-effective facility occupancy plan to be understood and accepted before a financial commitment was made. The new integrated computer system was established in the old facility to ensure tracking and cross-billing was possible **before** the occupancy. The staff saw the new facility as a benefit to the change process, and the significantly increased net income from the first day of occupancy made the doctors **very** happy.

The desire to control one's destiny does not always mean striving for the status quo. The desire to thrive means the desire to live a life rich in experiences and accomplishment. Practice number two made that happen for everyone, while practice number one feared sharing the dream and committing to the change.

The Business of Veterinary Program Planning

The first rule of budgeting—
the front door must swing.
—Dr. T.E. Catanzaro

From the above examples, the Introduction, and the Preface, it is evident that this new *management in transition* is moving from holding the status quo and *doing things right* to and understanding that veterinary practice is a business. The accounting approach to business planning is budgeting with cost control; this procedure is generally needed in the veterinary practice, but it is only effective for one or two cycles, until costs are controlled. The traditional veterinary methods of fiscal management are to beat the expense percentages to death when compared to the national averages (average is the best of the worst or the worst of the best—which do you want to be?). Veterinary-specific software systems generally tell you everything about income centers, but none are yet linked to any expense center comparisons. The accountant's system is to catalog your checks into as many categories as possible so the profit and loss (P&L) statement (income statement) looks impressive. However, note that sales is usually the **only** income category. Then you wonder why most veterinary practices do not have a dynamic budgeting process.

The Dynamic Budget Planning Process

When I refer to a dynamic budget planning process, I envision income centers that are matched to expense centers. The income and expense centers are similar to those shown in the AAHA Chart of Accounts published a decade and a half ago, but they are shown in greater, tailored, practice-specific detail. When I speak of significant ratios, I refer to expense compared to income for the same line item, to specific program income compared to outpatient visits, to fluid therapy units compared to general anesthetic cases, or even to diagnostic sales compared to pharmacy sales (by DVM and by practice). Let's try a test:

Question: The cost of goods sold for a companion animal practice is 18.3 percent of gross revenues for drugs and medical supplies, and another 2.5 percent of gross revenues for food sales; costs of laboratory/X-ray/ECG diagnostic services are 8.5 percent of gross revenues. Which percentage(s) appear inappropriately high or low?

Answer: Do not jump into this discussion with both feet until you know the rest of the story. Here are the income factors: Drugs and medical supplies brought in $375,000 in sales, food brought in $19,500, and laboratory/X-ray/ECG diagnostic services accounted for $98,500 of the practice gross. Total gross income was $985,400 for the period in this study. Now your answers would be

✓ Pharmacy sales were over two times expenses, so there is a good return based on the mark-up.

✓ For food, there is over $5,000 of product missing (even if we sold the food at cost); even maintenance diets should bring in about 25 percent net.

✓ The diagnostics only brought in about $15,000 net, a net income figure almost 10 times below expectations because the reported expenses were significantly higher than expected. Film and developing fluid, ECG paper and contact cream, outside laboratory costs, and reagents are low cost. Someone probably added equipment or maintenance to the wrong expense category.

Okay, so you feel I tricked you, but how often do you make a snap judgement on practice operations based on old habits, old information, or someone else's perspective (like those generalized articles in periodicals)? The focus must be on your practice, your community, and your clients if you want the front door to swing! A similar set of numbers exists for mixed animal practices, especially in farm-call pricing, mileage, and sale-barn fees, and when the practices compete with the "white truck" selling drugs up and down the back roads. A dynamic budget means we know how much money it took to create how much income within a specific practice program (dentistry, X-ray, laboratory, vaccinations, etc.).

Consider vaccinations. How many practices still hide their consultation fee from the client and charge $45 to $60 for the annual vaccination visit and exam? Why? Most of our consulting clients have started to use the term "doctor's consultation" on the invoice and on the telephone to differentiate the wellness examination by a paraprofessional staff member from a visit where the doctor is present and participates in discussions. This differentiation is critical when you exist in a community where other veterinarians, super pet stores, and vaccine clinics have made price a commodity to shop for in pet health care. I don't mind a 10-minute vaccine appointment with a paraprofessional for a wellness exam, but if clients want a doctor's consultation, they need to be scheduled for at least 20 minutes. The secret motivator is not that secret. The front door must swing for **any** program to be effective!

A dynamic budget process means we accept the forecast as targets, and if we hit the target we are okay. If we hit the bull's-eye every time, we are exceptional (and more likely, a falsifier of data). Each quarter, we look at what our in-service training plan did to affect specific programs and assess if the expense and income ratio changed based on the new knowledge shared within the team. If it did as expected, we must change the next quarter's budget to reflect the new trends and make new forecasts on lateral areas of interest. What does this mean in application? Please look at this simple example:

Issue: The practice decides it must start to use a *laboratory test waiver* before any general anesthesia for forensic reasons. It was added to the bottom of the *Surgery and Hospitalization Authorization Form* (from the AVMA Directory). The practice leadership decided to add a minimum level to the practice's existing over-six-years-old profile policy. [The basic profile was to include packed cell volume (PCV) and total protein (TP) (costing less than two dollars using only a hematocrit tube and a refractometer), plus a urine stick-screening test for BUN, for a charge of $9.50; the full profile was to include, in addition, the CBC and Chem Panel, for $45.50.] Each client would be asked to waive his/her animal's right to this screening so the practice could save the client money.

Results: Surprisingly, 60 percent of the owners of under-six-years-old pets opted for the basic $9.50 screen, and with the existing surgery pace, that brought in an additional $600 in sales (for a cost of $120) per month, or $1,800 for the quarter. To their utter astonishment, another 25 percent of the owners of under-six-years-old pets selected the full profile and made the practice an extra $1,000 monthly gross they had not expected ($3,000 per quarter). Since no one expected any impact, just a lot of waivers, the practice must now adjust the next quarter's projections. Where will the adjustments occur? In pre-anesthetic, of course, but what about the geriatric animal baseline laboratory profiles that were offered during annual exams only by exception in the past? In fact, the doctors became so comfortable with the increased client awareness of laboratory profiles that the senior friends program enabled many more over-six-years-old pets to receive baseline profiles. Slowly, in about a year, they started to offer baseline profiles when animals entered their adult stage of life, so there was a set of values to compare to when there was a crisis.

There are many applications of looking at the programs, such as having four levels of dental prophylaxis (1+, 2+, 3+, and 4+, based on the four pictures on the back of the CET brochure). The average single price for a dental visit should be the 2+ cost, and the mouth requiring more extensive treatment will have two more cost levels (where the 4+ cost is about twice the 2+ cost). Now the dentistry program can be priced and promoted to the client who takes good care of his/her pet's mouth, giving the client a price break based on the worst case scenario. Similarly, there can be four levels of bandaging (joint and bandage dependent) and four levels of hospitalization (o.d./b.i.d. to ICU). To keep the front door swinging, good clients must feel they are appreciated, and having levels of care allows them either recognition or options. Both are elements that will bring clients back to your practice, as well as encourage them to spread the word about their recognition.

There are many other programs that should be addressed, but each practice is limited by its past and by the vision of its leadership. The above are only examples of practice entry into program-based budgeting, but the examples have been taken from real-life veterinary practices. Clients must perceive a benefit when presented with two yes options (first introduced in the *Veterinary Forum* article, "Increasing Client Options—Changing the Way We Look at Office Calls," January 1993, 54–56). Satisfied clients make the front door swing! There are challenges to making this system work, and they must be addressed in the earliest development phases, either with your consultant's help or with strong personal beliefs and an individual vision.

Implementation of Program-based Planning

How do you get enough time to do all the new stuff needed for program-based planning? Simple. **You** don't. It must be a team effort. Every staff member must be involved in the new programs and processes. The leadership establishes clear core values, assigns accountability for reasonable outcomes, then becomes visionaries and trainers. The following six elements must be accepted as a minimum set of requirements and expectations for program-based budgeting to work:

• The practice must have a team that believes. They must believe in the core values of the practice and the standards of quality health-care delivery. As patient advocates, they must believe in the why of the programs, not see them as just new income sources for the boss.

- The leadership must be willing to train to trust. Each member of the staff must have the in-service training opportunity to gain confidence and competency in the new programs and the support procedures. A trusted staff member will receive an outcome accountability, and the doctor or manager will not worry, or even care, about the process. Success measurements will be founded in outcomes and results.

- The practice leadership will practice daily the three **R**s of building self-worth in **all** the staff members: **R**espect, **R**esponsibility, and **R**ecognition. Respect for all immediately, responsibility concurrent with training to trust, and recognition, since behavior rewarded is behavior repeated.

- Be ready to change every habit and modify every new program to respond to community needs. Strategic response replaces the outdated strategic planning process. Be ready to do unique and unusual things as if they were usual and do the usual in a new and unusual way. Continuous quality improvement (CQI) means **every** staff member is accountable for unilaterally causing improvement and change on a regular basis for the benefit of the client, the staff, or the practice entity.

- Be ready to track more things, specific to programs, based on procedures as well as dollars. Be ready to upgrade computer knowledge and increase trend assessment discussions within the staff. Start getting balanced financial reports. Pair income to expense centers, with expenses listed in order of importance rather than alphabetized. Be ready to change accountants if the firm will not support your effort. Be ready to have every member initiate new programs and target actions every quarter. Embrace practice performance planning rather than the performance appraisals of the past.

- Accept the fact that this is a new practice process, not a gimmick or new program. Once started, you can't go back. Once started, you are committed to change the future, forever. Change will be the norm, and if a particular program or practice seems okay, it hasn't been assessed well enough for adaptation to the future.

VETERINARY PRACTICE CHECKLIST FOR SELF-ASSESSMENT

(Please circle the number, or assign a mid-point number.)

1. Does your current invoicing system allow efficient preparation and printing?

Yes	=	0
No	=	10
Not important to us	=	2

2. Does your current system allow close tracking of receivables?

Yes, easily	=	0
Not close enough	=	4
Not important to us	=	6
Not easily	=	8
No	=	10

3. Does your current system automate monthly client billing?

Yes, easily	=	0
Not important to us	=	2
Yes, but with difficulty	=	5
No	=	10

4. Can your current system change client message based on aging of accounts?

Yes, easily and automatically	=	0
With close personal effort	=	5
No	=	10

5. Does your current system allow you to manage cash flow and payables?

Yes, easily and automatically	=	0
With close personal effort	=	5
Takes substantial analysis to maintain	=	8
Not managed well	=	10

6. Are you on an automated vendor check printing system?

Yes, easily and automatically	=	0
With close personal effort	=	5
No	=	10

7. Does you current system maintain a perpetual balance inventory?

Yes, easily and automatically	=	0
With close personal effort	=	5
No	=	10

8. Are client estimates an automated process?

Yes, easily and automatically	=	0
With close personal effort	=	5
No	=	10

9. Do the end-of-month financial reports match income centers to expense centers?

Yes, easily and automatically	=	0
With close personal effort	=	5
No	=	10

10. Does it take extensive staff training time to learn the tracking systems?

No, easy and automated system	=	0
Not much; procedures are keyed to recurring reports	=	4
With multiple recycling	=	6
Yes	=	10

11. Are end-of-month financial reports generated in-house?

Yes, easily and automatically	=	0
With close personal effort	=	5
No	=	10

12. Does the accountant convert the cash-based program data to tax-based data?

Yes, easily and automatically	=	0
Yes, quarterly, with our guidance	=	4
Annually, with close personal effort	=	7
No	=	10

System Flexibility Issues

1. Have you modified the professions Chart of Accounts to meet your own needs?

Yes	=	0
Use them unchanged	=	3
We use one from our accountant	=	6
We don't have a system	=	10

2. Do your current tracking systems change with the practice's evolution?

Yes, easily	=	0
No	=	10

3. Can your current system develop customized reports to track trends?

    Yes, easily and automatically   =   0

    With close personal effort   =   5

    No   =   10

4. Is your word processing integrated with a spread sheet system?

    Yes, easily and automatically   =   0

    Separate programs, manual combining   =   5

    No   =   10

5. Are you willing to change computer systems or add accounting software?

    Yes   =   0

    Yes, but not happily   =   4

    Only if you can prove a major cost benefit   =   8

    No   =   10

Networking Concerns

1. Are you on the Internet for veterinary computerized resource access?

    Yes, VIN or NOAH (or both)   =   0

    Yes, but not for clinical exchanges   =   4

    No   =   10

2. Do you use a management review system for your practice operational data?

    Yes, practice consultant   =   0

    Yes, 20s-type group   =   4

    Yes, regionalized   =   6

    Yes, with a close friend   =   8

    No   =   10

3. Is your accountant monitoring the practice data against national trends?

    Yes   =   0

    Yes, but only when we provide it   =   4

    No   =   10

4. Do you use a management/leadership team to review the practice program data?

    Yes, informally monthly and formally quarterly =   0

    Yes, but not routinely   =   4

    No   =   10

5. Does the management/leadership team have staff members represented?

Yes, informally and formally	=	0
Yes, but not routinely	=	4
No	=	10

Reporting System

1. How long does it take after the close of the month to complete the reports?

10 staff hours or less	=	0
10–40 staff hours	=	5
11–40 doctor hours	=	8
We don't do it	=	10

2. Would you prefer that a supporting organization compile reports?

Yes, with practice-specific contract	=	0
Yes, but as a group	=	4
No	=	10

3. Does the monthly tracking system effectively track tax and benefit issues?

Yes, informally monthly and formally quarterly	=	0
Yes, but not routinely	=	4
No	=	10

4. Do you have an annual budget?

Yes, program-based	=	0
Yes, expense-based	=	5
Yes, but not routinely used	=	8
No	=	10

5. Does the monthly tracking feed the practice's program planning process?

Yes, informally monthly and formally quarterly	=	0
Yes, but not routinely	=	4
No	=	10

QUANTITATIVE SCORING

50 points or less—Your current system puts your veterinary practice into the top 10 percent. You may want to hire an administrator who is a trusted management specialist to quantify the excellent track record. You may also want to contact a consultant to fine-tune your system or take it to the next level, but the consultant should have an integrated, people-based approach. You crunch your numbers well!

51–100 points—Your current system is not grossly obsolete, and you are still securely in the top half of the veterinary practices (above average). The need for a good hospital manager (CVPM) or administrator for getting a better handle on the operations without taking doctors away from patient care and client-centered activities is evident. There may be upgrades that can assist your practice; this practice is a good candidate for fine-tuning assistance for a veterinary-exclusive, program-centered, consulting group, if the personalities match with the practice team.

101–150 points—You have an average practice (average = best of the worst or worst of the best). This means program planning is probably not operating effectively, and program-budget systems are not well integrated. A hospital manager is needed to add a monitoring system and a human resource advocate to the operations. With the help of a consultant to assist in the realignment of duties and the integration of the manager, you can fine-tune your system or take it to the next level; the consultant and manager must have an integrated, people-based, program-heavy approach so you can make money while changing.

151–200 points—Your current system is most likely inadequate to keep pace with the changing demands of this profession. Problems are likely to overtake you and add frustration (burnout). If you cannot afford a practice manager right now, start working with a consultant so you can; you should ensure the consultant is willing to start growing a manager internally, and not build an umbilical cord of high cost, "forever" support systems (although this option is indicated in a few practices where the leadership cannot trust a manager). Also, start shopping for both a consultant and manager to expand your alternatives right now.

201 points or more—To score this high, your current system would have to be almost nonexistent. This means a major practice philosophy change, more team work, and a new look at the future vision of the practice leadership. The practice manager entering this system will not be able to solve all the issues alone; outside expertise will be needed to reverse dysfunctional habits. The consultant you select (since your score proves you can't do it yourself) must be able to (1) integrate the programs through the manager(s) with training and nonthreatening tracking techniques, (2) have veterinary profession-specific experience, (3) provide a mentorship to your multifaceted team, to support your efforts and mission focus, and (4) convince you that change is critical for survival.

Note: If your score exceeds 100 points, a veterinary-specific consulting group should be added to your research list of potential practice business resources. The web page <www.v-p-c.com> has the most recent, unbiased, opinion survey of over 40 nationally recognized veterinary practice consultants (the Veterinary Consultant's Network [VCN] modified Delphi study) and provides guidelines of what to review and seek when searching for a veterinary practice consultant.

- The VCN lists provide insight to the characteristics to seek when searching for the consultant(s) who can tailor veterinary programs to practice personalities and practice philosophies.

- A diverse team of business consultants, willing to become **your** team, can be far more beneficial than some of the recently emerging outsiders to our profession.

- A good, veterinary-exclusive consultant can train your banker, attorney, and accountant as well as your manager.

- Beware of the cookbook, guaranteed solutions (stated before the team or community is assessed), those that just tell you to discount or jack up your fees, and one-deep veterinary consulting firms.

2 Governance

Governance is not just a political term—it is a new form of management for affiliations and mergers.
—Dr. T.E. Catanzaro

ASSOCIATIONS NEED GOVERNANCE

It should be self-evident that every veterinary association, national, state, or local, needs to understand governance, yet this is an invalid assumption. Many associations have board members who try to direct the affiliated voluntary organization as they direct their own practices. The difference is significant, and governance acuity affects participation and membership renewals.

In veterinary medicine, governance, and even the concept of governing boards, is alien, but in human health care it has existed from the very beginning of cooperative time. The client's need for quality health care and the technology for delivering the best of care creates a core of functions that each modern veterinary hospital must serve. In small private practices, governance and ownership are synonymous, but in affiliated or merged veterinary healthcare delivery situations a new structure is needed. Emergency practice boards have generally been the first introduction of veterinarians to the responsibilities of governance. The term *governance* describes the relationship between a board of directors and a CEO, between a hospital board and the hospital administrator, or between the operations committee of an emergency practice and the VECCS-certified emergency clinic director. The role of governance is always evolving and takes many forms, but some things remain constant:

- The *basic argument* usually can be summarized by the question, "How much influence does the governance board have on daily operations?"

- The *basic complaint* by staff is: "Why don't they give us enough resources (people, money, equipment) so we can do our job?"

- The *basic blaming statement* is usually something akin to, "They don't understand all the pressures and demands being made on us!"

Now that the negatives are on the table, let's move forward and try to understand the manager's role in this newly evolving structure. Let's look at some basic veterinary healthcare systems today that require a governance structure:

- The shareholder-owned emergency practice, briefly mentioned above.

- The corporate practice where the owners are either too many or residing elsewhere.

- The central inpatient hospital owned by many outlying outpatient facility owners.

- Professional affiliations, such as multiple specialty practices under one roof with some common use areas. For these, governance is the **only** way to keep the participants in some type of stable core values or philosophy position when assessing resource allocations.

- Buying coops, veterinary medical associations, and other membership-type affiliations. These have always had a governance (board) structure, but board members are seldom trained in governance.

Why do we need to make an issue of governance in a text on managers in transition? The three main reasons are listed below:

- A governance board **requires** an administrator for daily operations and implementation decisions, just like any set of shareholders needs a board (executive/operations committee) for policy and direction decisions.

- A manager must become a leader to work with a governance board, and these boards will **increase** in the new millennium (review the structures listed above for a reality check); the exceptional managers will become healthcare administrators in the future of veterinary medicine.

- Governance is written about regularly in human health care because it is a constantly evolving operational need of hospitals, but no one has ever written about it in veterinary medicine—welcome to the new millennium!

ANOTHER ASSOCIATION INSIGHT

In veterinary associations, administrators are often called executive directors. These executive directors are the true unsung heroes of organized veterinary medicine. A board that embraces the tenants of governance makes life easier for the executive director and the association staff, and the association becomes more responsive to the members and programs of the affiliation.

In reality, while often combined in smaller veterinary practices, there are six basic systems in most every veterinary healthcare organizational structure: the governing system, the executive operational system, the healthcare delivery systems, the planning and marketing systems for community outreach, the financial system, and the information systems. The governance system must be the one system accountable for making the other five systems look good, both internally, from within the organizational structure, and externally, to the community.

The Functions of Governance

Society has established, through laws and traditions, two basic criteria for the actions of governance boards. First, their actions must be prudent and reasonable (rather than simply well-intentioned or successful). Board members should be careful, thoughtful, and judicious in decision making; they need not always be right. Second, since board members hold a position of trust for the owners of the facility; they must not take unfair advantage of their membership, and they must, to the best of their ability, direct their actions to the benefit of the whole ownership. In for-profit veterinary systems, this means avoiding situations that give special advantage to some participants, particularly the directors themselves (e.g., requiring all radiology referrals to access the facility radiologist through another service first).

In human health care, governance has undergone many changes and has had many formats. Consensus on the best system has eluded even the most skilled of healthcare administrators, since variances between for-profit and not-for-profit and variations in community demographics, fiscal structuring, provider affiliation, and system interrelationships cause each situation to be different, sometimes slightly, and other times radically. As a consulting firm, we have experienced the same wide environmental and staff variances in veterinary medicine. Many governance boards start with a list of elements that can be done best by the individual members, then as they mature in cooperation, they expand their charter with a list of things they think they can do best. With the most successful governance boards, they begin their list with those activities that **only** they can do.

In the written and oral exams for diplomates of the American College of Healthcare Executives, one of the 10 areas of certification is governance; there are common themes, with little or no disagreement, on the essential functions of governance:

- To select and sanction the hospital administrator.

- To establish the mission focus, vision, and core values for operational decisions.

- To review strategic community and facility decisions on a recurring basis.

- To approve the annual program-based budget, including the establishment of equitable lease allocation agreements with the tenants.

- To resolve boundary disputes and monitor other conflict resolution actions.

- To credential services and members of the professional staff.

- To monitor system performance against plans and budgets.

While the structure, authority, and operational integrity of governance varies, the following areas are monitored within any governance system:

- *Trustee or governing board.* The board concept is an old and essential part of human hospitals. When hospitals have tried to dispense with the governance board concept, within six months they have had to redefine and rebuild the governance board for conflict resolution and hospital survival planning. The board's functional role has evolved toward boundary spanning, identification of exchange opportunities, and strategic assessment of community trends and demands. The board's planning emphasis has moved away from daily operational issues to a broader and more generalized policy and precedent function, including establishing the core values for making tough decisions.

- *Executive system.* The position of president and chief executive officer in early human healthcare facilities becomes that of the hospital administrator in veterinary medical facilities. The term *executive system* actually includes the functions of a centralized management support team for the facility as well as those of the implementation agent for the policy and precedent parameters set by the governance board. This executive administrative team not only provides day-to-day operational support for all tenants and credentialed professionals/services operating within the facility, but also supports the needs of the governance system.

- *Medical staff.* Although the functions of the medical staff are clinical, the nature of the contract between the staff members and the organization as a whole is a critical governance activity. What began as open staff almost a century ago gave way to closed staff between the first and second world wars, and became privileged staff in the mid-1970s. Quality reviews were made increasingly rigorous through the post-war decades, enforced by a peer utilization review process. In veterinary medicine, this is a governance board issue, and the utilization review of professionals and services is called the *credentialing* process. In some larger veterinary hospitals, a chief of professional services (CPS) is added to the executive system to act as liaison between the governance board and the professional staff.

- *Planning and marketing system.* Well-managed community hospitals did not start rudimentary market niche planning until the mid-1970s, when federal legislation resulted in concerns about cost and equitable access. Healthcare promotions have evolved to establishing a market niche within the community, which means assessing, evaluating, influencing and responding to exchange opportunities, not unlike the veterinary specialty hospitals serving the general practices in the area or region. The cost control associated with economy of scale operations fosters a more aggressive strategic planning position being developed concurrently with any marketing concept.

- *Public relations and relationships.* In the broadest sense, public relations includes not-for-profit fund raising in some animal welfare facilities, but it is also a critical function for specialty hospitals (including emergency and critical care facilities) trying to influence referrals from general practices. Promotion of services, which is part of marketing, includes both advertising and public relations. In simplest terms, the way the practice or institution is perceived by its exchange partners is heavily influenced by its public relations/relationship system. It is therefore essential to monitor this system to ensure that it contributes to both operational growth and increased utilization of fiscal assets for better liquidity.

- *Information management.* Information arises from the activities of three major areas: finance, healthcare delivery, and governance. Data from these three sources becomes available at unequal rates, but the information provided by each and the interrelationships among them are essential to the decision-making process. There are both open and closed system requirements, due to the confidentiality of client/patient information, the segregation of function for fiscal matters, and the forensic liability associated with drugs and veterinary healthcare delivery. In larger veterinary facilities, information management often becomes an operational function of the hospital administrator and an information service coordinator.

There are many operational systems concurrently functioning with any veterinary facility, including client relations, patient admission and disposition (PAD), finance, clinical specialties, medical care, clinical support services, nursing care, human resource management, the physical plant, central medical supply (CMS), and other related activities. These are day-to-day operations entrusted to the hospital administrator and the executive team. The governance board seldom gets involved in any of these except for initial credentialing and mediation of those boundary issues associated with interservice relationships that cannot be resolved between the facility occupants (and may result in decredentialing).

The New Era for Veterinary Medicine

As we closed the books on the twentieth century, the vast majority of our consulting practice had been shifting from management to leadership; we were going into veterinary practices of many sizes, species, and organizational structures and facilitating team restructuring projects, including

- Streamlining operations and looking at affiliations or mergers,

- Resolving conflicts between practice staff and professional elements,

- Addressing the economy of scale (e.g., implementing high-density scheduling),

- Repositioning practices to better meet community demands,

- Reorganizing management and clinical operations by staff members,

- Implementing quarterly performance planning rather than annual retrospective appraisals, and

- Enhancing programs and procedures, based on the core values of the practice leadership.

While we have published many leadership and veterinary management texts in the past three years, we suddenly found that we had done only about two-thirds of the leadership reorganization needed for the new millennium. Veterinary practices were merging, the number of specialty hospitals was increasing, and public corporate practices were emerging without a proven management structure; but new management roles had not yet evolved. Veterinary medicine is truly a profession in evolution, but a revolution is required in most growing practices to break the tradition of doctor control and expand the affiliated and administrative roles of staff.

As you assess the environment in which you think governance review may be required, assess the following factors:

- Representative governance is often a barrier to change.
    - ✓ Players often resist change rather than lead it.
    - ✓ The traditionalists are the caboose versus the engine of the train.
    - ✓ Leadership needs to be accepted as change revolution.
    - ✓ Management is seen as stability and status quo (death).

- Share the mission focus with the staff: it must be believed.
  - ✓ A mission focus defines the **core business** of the **practice systems** and **how** the practice philosophy is applied to every day activities.
  - ✓ A mission focus helps make difficult decisions.
  - ✓ The mission focus is based on the core values of the board.
  - ✓ Core values are inviolate, even for the board members.

- Prevention of bad data.
  - ✓ Only Congress believes we can be taxed into prosperity.
  - ✓ Expense-based decisions often cause stagnation (and death).
  - ✓ Reinvestment in the future is a fiscal commitment to action.
  - ✓ Program-based decisions require expense centers and income centers to be matched business entities.
  - ✓ Data is raw; information is made relational for decision-making purposes.

- Attention to deadwood.
  - ✓ Attention to process and bylaws does not mean control of operations.
  - ✓ Personnel must have confidence in each other's behavior.
  - ✓ The board needs methods and criteria for board reorganization.
  - ✓ Conflicts of interest are never permitted.
  - ✓ No independent authority is held by any team member.
  - ✓ The board can and **must** remove an employee for cause.

- Job description of board members.
  - ✓ Members must focus on the big picture.
  - ✓ Responsibilities must be based on mission focus.
  - ✓ Assigned tasks must not be centered in details.
  - ✓ Commitment to the practice entity is a requirment for holding office.
  - ✓ Strategic assessment replaces operational guidance as the job focus.

- A board meeting agenda is required.
  - ✓ The agenda must be available one year in advance for strategic issues.
  - ✓ There is no killing the cash cow without replacement stock.
  - ✓ There is no protecting the cash cow if it has outlived its usefulness.

      ✓ Unscheduled issues are tabled until the next meeting.

      ✓ Strategic response is community-centered, not practice-centered.

Barriers to Effective Governance: The Seven Deadly Sins

Expanding the affiliation interaction and administrative roles of staff often requires a new board structure and function, as well as a new operational mentality focused on we rather than me. In the majority of the group-based organizations we have worked with, the people involved in governance roles have not known their own structure. When talking to the chair of an emergency or specialty group, you find that the core values, mission, and vision of the combined organization have seldom been addressed; in this situation, the organizational leadership makes decisions based on the values of the individual practice representative(s). This format is often based on turf protection rather than community needs, and decisions and strategic responses are made based on the benefits to board or committee members, rather than on benefits to the combined organization. And the real issues get lost or ignored in the shuffle.

The thesis we normally take, when we consider the issue of governance, is that governance really needs to be the engine that pulls the train of change for the veterinary healthcare organization. Very frequently, in America today, committees and boards are the caboose dragging along behind, and frequently the caboose has the brakes on. Boards are not only eluding the process of change; they are actually the major resistant barrier to the effective implementation of change. What are boards supposed to do? What is their structure? How can we streamline them? We think examining these questions will go a long way toward moving organizations to where they need to be.

Let's look at some of the classic barriers in governance; we call them the seven deadly sins of ineffective governance.

1. Representational Governance

Representational governance is the most classic structural mechanism for forming group specialty systems; we often do not have alternatives in the beginning. In this structure, the board specifically or implicitly represents the subconstituent interest groups. The result is a system board composed of one-service-one-vote overseeing the facility, separate services, and boundary-issue decisions. It works reasonably well when you are making easy decisions. When the group must make tough decisions, the negative side of representational governance rears its ugly head. Often, as soon as a challenging situation arises, board members, instead of speaking for the best interests of the system as a whole, start thinking, what is in the best interest of my subgroup, my constituent group, or my suborganization. There are two ways to avoid this:

- Clarify roles and responsibilities and establish job descriptions and operational expectations for all board members.

- When facilitating functional governance, put a great amount of energy into the removal-for-cause provisions, including such factors as meeting attendance, loyalty, maintaining confidentiality, and decision support. The debates that precede a decision must be retired with the vote, and total support of the decision is **required** of all board members **all** the time.

2. Lack of Mission Focus

The second great sin of ineffective governance is lack of mission focus. Boards who don't have a shared understanding of what the organization is attempting to do cannot facilitate the appropriate outcomes. Let's assume that each individual member of your current board has a different understanding of the purpose of the organization; each has a different implicit idea of the **real** mission of the organization. The group has a tremendous difficulty, because they will make inconsistent and unpredictable decisions, which paradoxically, will alienate the very stakeholders they are trying to integrate. So one of the fundamental characteristics of effective governance is that the board has an agreed upon belief system or principle-based foundation for decision making that is equally and consistently applied in all situations. This belief system is not based on what individual members believe is right or wrong; it is based on what the group as a whole believes is right or wrong. An effective board uses its foundation core values, vision, and mission focus as the basis of their decision making.

As a part of establishing an agreed upon belief system, boards compose mission statements. Although many mission statements look beautiful, they often are pabulum on a piece of paper.

- What is the definition of a good mission statement? A good mission statement helps you make difficult decisions. Take the three or four most difficult decisions that your organization has made in the last couple of years or project the most challenging decisions that you think your organization will face in the next four or five years, and consult the mission statement for guidance. If the mission statement, more often than not, does not give you guidance, it is not meaningful.

- A clear mission focus helps you make difficult decisions, and it helps the board make consistent decisions. So we have two format issues for governance: (1) many boards have not spent the required time defining a meaningful mission focus, and (2) boards that have established a focus do not use the core values in their decision-making process and thus start to develop an implicit mission. The most common implicit deviations from the mission are personal survival and financial viability. So although you may see the written mission care of the community, the implicit mission is financial viability. This type of implicit mission generates inconsistency and unpredictability and is usually signaled by high staff turnover.

3. Resistance to Change

Resistance to change is probably the biggest obstacle to effective governance that we confront; it is the tendency of boards to resist change rather than to lead it. This is a great problem because in an environment of revolutionary change, the concepts and roles of leadership change as well. In periods of great stability and incremental change, such as those we are leaving behind, the role of leadership was fundamentally to keep things as they had been, to maintain stability and predictability. Most veterinarian-based oversight groups try to ensure that the process of change is not too disorienting or disruptive and that it is incremental. This is called the committee form of reference in most professional associations. In periods of revolutionary change, where we are now, the past is no predictor of future success. Where you can't make linear predictions based on what happened yesterday or on what is happening today, the role of the leader is not to maintain the status quo or ensure comfort, it is to facilitate the process of change. One way of addressing this problem is to adjust the board composition. So we recommend that a combined specialty practice add a member from the local VMA executive board or that an emergency practice add a member from the local humane society (these are safe members **if** the board job description and mission focus are a charter for each board member). Another mechanism is to push forward with the need to create the future, but this is very frightening because this model of leadership requires the board to anticipate what is going to happen and to start changes before they are needed. Suddenly the board becomes the agent of change rather than the friend of the status quo. The fundamental dynamic of this leadership model is to break the mold of complacency and to create tension. And this board role creates almost an adversarial relationship.

THE CORTEZ STORY

Cortez was sent by the Queen of Spain to take over Central and South America. He landed with his several dozen ships and several hundred ragged conquistadors to take over the natives. Cortez was ready, but his men said, "Wait a minute, there is a civilization here: millions of Aztecs, Toltecs, and Mayans. We can't do this. Lets go home." Cortez gave them a rousing speech, but they said, "Wonderful speech, but we are going home—if you get in our way, we'll kill you." Cortez realized he had to make the men think that they would have their way, while still accomplishing his mission. So he said, "We'll go home, but we can't go home empty handed. There is a little village over the hill. Let's go pillage it and take whatever we can find, so we won't go back empty handed. We'll go home and say that is all there was, that the trip wasn't worth it." His men agreed. Then Cortez added, "I'm just getting over being seasick from crossing the Atlantic, and I'm not really that hot to get back on the ship today; since we brought enough stores with us for several months, let's take the wine and have a party." After he got them all on the beach, they drank all the wine, and to cap the party, he then burned the ships. Turning to his men, Cortez said, "What are we going to do now?" The men looked at him and said, "Guess we're going to take over Central and South America, you son of … ." With a little help from smallpox, they did it. After they had been successful and had accomplished more than their objectives, Cortez turned to his men and, in the classic failing of leadership, said, "I told you so. I knew we could do it." The men responded as expected and killed him. That is the trap of leadership in terms of facilitating the process of change.

When you look at history, you see that leaders who have brought their governments or their countries through great periods of disruption are often dumped after the disruption is over. That's why England did not reelect Winston Churchill following World War II, and that is one of the reasons I suspect the United States did not reelect George Bush following the Gulf War. We say, "That was great, thanks very much, get out now, we're done." This is a very different model of leadership for boards to get comfortable with, and unfortunately most veterinarians, when confronted with this role, tend to back away from it. That is why most veterinary boards interpret their role as maintaining stability, being forestallers rather than agents of change. This perception creates a dam effect: if your actions keep changes away, the longer you keep them away, the more the force builds up, so that when they come, they come with an almost irresistible force and sweep everything away. So reeducation is needed:

- The board says everyone needs to change: Management, the doctors, and the staff need to change, but the board is going to stay the same. We are going to keep the same structure, get the same information, and have the same people on the board we've always had. This pattern is typically seen as a board's reluctance to change itself. The pattern is changed by redefining the playing field (mission focus, core values, vision statement, job descriptions, etc.).

- Governance is often one of the last vestiges of resistance to change that we see in health care. The agents of governance must confront themselves and ask, "Where is the logic to this resistance?" Interestingly, most will recognize that resistance is fairly illogical, but they are emotionally unwilling to change. In many cases some consulting group gets hired to be the outside agent of change.

4. Bad Governance Information

One of the reasons boards succumb to the ineffective governance practices is that they are getting bad governance information. They are getting old style, process-oriented, warmed-over management reports—information that forces them to monitor what has happened as opposed to focusing on the future. They are getting information that is focused on hospital inpatient activities, when most all of the real business is coming from outside sources. It is very common to see a disconnection between the data that a board gets and the stated strategy of the organization. This is one of the classic barriers to effective governance, which is again based on a poorly understood mission focus. To escape this pitfall, consider the following:

- The executive group needs to change raw data into information before the board gets the paper. There must be a major emphasis centered on external forces (e.g., referral rates from general practices).

- When addressing internal issues, the board must address hospital policies from a general oversight perspective, looking at boundary issues, as well as addressing the strategic positioning of the complex.

5. Failure to Dump Deadwood

Another classic sin is failure to dump the deadwood from the board. Firing their own members is one task that most boards avoid like the plague. A progressive board charter includes both a mechanism for removing a board member from office midterm and the criteria for doing so. Think about the bylaws of the board.

- The board bylaws need to communicate to every member of the board that the organization is what matters, that the board represents the system, and that the board does not play around with the mission focus or core values. Many people on boards don't understand that the role of a board, fundamentally, is to operate as a cohesive group and that individual board members have no independent authority. There are veterinary board members who feel that if they do not agree with a particular board decision, it is their duty to work against it. That is not the case. When an issue has been debated, the board has voted, and you find yourself in the minority, there are only two choices, even if you feel passionately about the issue. You must either support the vote of the board or resign.

- If a dissenting board member remains on the board and either works against any vote or constantly reintroduces the vote, the board should correct the member's behavior. If the board doesn't, board performance is fractured; in the absence of board action, cliques will form, and we will see kind of a death spiral of board function.

- Boards need to create a culture of performance and accountability. No one is allowed to join the board unless they are willing to meet these performance criteria characteristics. Criteria address the basics: violation of conflict of interest or confidentiality policies, meeting attendance, and full support of board votes.

- If a board member is not coming to the meetings, violating the conflict of interest parameters, or ignoring any of the decisions of the board, that member should be off the board. Criteria must also address qualitative issues: thoughtful participation, reviewing the agenda materials before board meetings, not being a one-issue participant, not subverting the work of the board, etc.

- Boards should also have term limits, and there should be no auto-matic renewal at the end of a term. For example, if a three-year term is established and members are allowed to serve a maximum of three consecutive three-year terms, no one is guaranteed to serve on the board for nine years. During and after the first term there is evalua-tion against the criteria. If the member has met performance criteria A, B, C, and D, and if his/her skill sets are still needed on the board, then the member will be invited back. In most practices establishing a governance board for the first time, we like to stagger the initial terms: one-third of the board members have a one-year term, one-third have a two-year term, and one-third have a three-year term. Subsequent board members, by election or selection, serve a three-year term of board service. In this way, there is a continuity of knowledge and a maturation of the board understanding of mem-bers over their three-year terms.

6. Holding On to the Past

Maintaining cumbersome, outmoded, governance structures is an-other sin of ineffective governance. Winston Churchill said, "First we create our structures, then they create us." Many traditional veterinary governance structures add costs to the system without adding value. Consider how the board can ensure that value is added.

- A recurring assessment of how much time the governance structure takes is essential. How much of an administrator's time is spent preparing for, attending, and following up on board and board com-mittee meetings? Any portion over 20 percent should be a warning signal. We've seen it as high as 78 percent; the manager's time was spent preparing for, attending, and following up on board meetings; talking to shareholders (who all considered themselves directors); at-tending meetings; and answering individual inquiries from share-holders. We regarded this as adding a tremendous amount of cost for very little value. To solve this problem, we introduced an elected three-person operations committee, accountable for governance and administrator oversight, called them directors, and reverted the re-maining shareholders to a hands-off, fiscal-based, pool of potential directors, elected at a rate of one per year.

- The board must create value in their decisions, which accounts for the external focus on client satisfaction and access. In the case of emergency hospitals, combined specialty hospitals, and other referral hospitals, the primary clients are referring veterinarians, general practices in the area, and in some cases, brood mare farms, or even horse trainers at large facilities, but **not** the animal owner. This is why timely referral letters, interservice harmony, and **never** bad mouthing a referring agent are considered boundary issues for governance.

7. Lack of Job Descriptions

Job descriptions are a very important factor in effective governance. You don't have to be a genius to figure out that a group that does not know what its job is won't do it very well. I am constantly struck by the fact that when you ask board members what the job of the board is, you get different answers from each person. There is no common understanding of what the board is supposed to do. This lays the foundation for a lack of strategic alignment as the board members go in different directions. Consider the importance of a clear and unified focus:

- Failure to understand the core business of the organization occurs as a specialist moves from being a knowledge broker providing services to acute individuals to being a service providing healthcare support to general practices scattered through an increasingly disparate community and the core business begins to change. The inability of any specialist to overcome the "me" paradigm makes turf wars and governance intervention inevitable.

- The board is the keeper of the core business; it focuses the organization's resources on the mission. If a board doesn't understand this, there will be serious problems. Operations committees that have been formed with the implicit purpose of protecting their favorite pieces of the system are an example of a classic barrier to change. A variation of this mind-set is the inability of the advocates of cash cows to accept a system-focused strategy. It is very difficult to get people who feel they are governing from a representational perspective to embrace mission-focused leadership during a period of change and be willing to take the dollars being generated from businesses today to invest in growing the veterinary businesses of tomorrow.

- Many of the veterinary healthcare systems we work with are composed of individuals who came from residency and academic environments (the epitome of not-for-profit operations). They carry not-for-profit paradigms like the Holy Grail, and they basically think that the purpose of the system is to maintain and enhance their clinical skill set. They don't realize that the fundamental characteristic of a system is that no one piece of a system is any more important than the system as a whole. Every piece of a system exists to enhance the system as a whole, and pieces of the system can be sacrificed or expanded, as necessary, to meet the strategy of the system.

Controlling the Chaos of Change

The inability of board members to understand the new millennium, emerging veterinary demands, or even the new healthcare environment, can be a major factor in maintaining liquidity for each and every participant in the system. Now what does this mean? It means, very simply, that there are two big areas a board must address. The board members must know the big picture, and they must trust others to know the details and submit summaries to the board on a quarterly basis. Concurrently, the definition of a good board member is someone who has a life outside veterinary medicine. What do I mean by that? Most veterinarians, on boards or running their own practice, do not look full of joy. As professionals, these veterinarians are spending 60 hours a week working, 20 hours a week reading, and 15 hours a week talking to people to figure out what the heck is going on in the community or with client access rates.

Too often we find a board that is dysfunctional due to micromanagement, either because they don't understand the big picture or because when trying to understand the big picture they get frightened. Such boards focus on the details, not because the details are critical, but because the details occupy their time to the exclusion of the big picture questions; this is the activity level trap. The board feels good because they are doing something, but what they are doing isn't the big picture–oriented stuff that needs to be done. Consequently, we find board members who are relatively sophisticated when it comes to veterinary economics averages and the details of the organization, but don't have a very good concept about what is likely to happen in their environment in four or five years. These board members don't have the ability to go out and create the future.

Refocusing boards on the big picture requires appropriate initial structuring as well as training development in making tough decisions on strategic issues. It also requires changing the information they get; this is a very important strategy for overcoming the micromanagement barrier. This problem is also addressed by the mission focus and personal job descriptions, which reduce ambiguity in roles and responsibilities. Every board runs into the issue of who does what, who bears the ultimate responsibility for which issues, and what the distinction is between what I do and what you do. To reduce some of these difficulties, we present a half-dozen tenets of tenacity when we establish the initial expectations of a board.

TENETS OF TENACITY

1. There are officers within the board, they are internally selected each year, and their job descriptions are supplemental to the board member job description.
2. Agenda issues are identified on an annual plan, with the tough ones being programmed for one per meeting, and they are addressed first at each meeting. These issues are tasked in advance to specific board member(s) who research the issue, apply the core values and mission focus, and insert no less than three key evaluation factors in the pre-published agenda, for board members to use in preparation for the meeting.
3. A sequential list of motions is maintained, and issues that have come up for vote are not reintroduced for vote within the following 11 months.
4. When any form of arbitrary turf statement is identified by any Board member, the issue will be tabled and tasked to an impartial board member task force for agenda evaluation (see tenet 2 above).
5. Confidentiality is a right and compromise an expectation; caring counts. Cooperation is required for harmony and system enhancement.
6. Board loyalty includes respect for individuals, services, and decisions (votes, existing policy, executive team, etc.). Failure to show respect can be cause for censure, removal from the board, or even decredentialing within the system if the offense is considered detrimental to the image or the moral or legal position of the system.

Governance for the Twenty-first Century

Engineering Veterinary Boards for a New Era

To get started on the correct tone, a new governance board must identify the core values of the affiliation, establish a facility-based mission focus, develop a clear vision of the veterinary healthcare delivery direction required for success, and then create a long-range plan. This is a repetitive process of goal setting, assessment, adjustment, and achievement. The veterinary governance board is striving for three ideal conditions to evolve:

- The goals of the affiliated organization, as a whole, are those that the larger community of referring veterinarians will appreciate and reward.

- Each unit or service of the affiliation has readily observable objectives that are consistent with the goals of the organization as a whole and that are available within the resources of the unit or service.

- The process of assessment and adjustment is carried out in a way that maximizes achievement of those goals and objectives.

No organization ever achieves the ideal. Good organizations are competitive on all three conditions, and continued success requires frequent attention to all three areas. The board is involved in the entire review process. The well-managed affiliated service hospital, however, has a governance board that focuses its attention on the initial steps of identifying core values, setting the mission and vision, and setting policies that will improve the consistency and efficacy of the overall process. To help start this process, three elements are critical to establishing an explicit mission focus for any affiliated group of veterinary healthcare professionals:

- *Community.* In most cases, this is a community of general practitioners, which cause animal owners and animals to access a specific level of specialized health care. For the board, it includes geographic, demographic, religious, and financial groups within the catchment area (this is variable, but is based on the scope of services, the available technology, and personal relationships).

- *Service.* Clinical specialists may be board-certified experts, but they are dependent upon the benefit awareness of referring veterinarians for their clients. Affiliations that center on developing a successful environment for their referral-based practices get to provide more services than those specialists who focus only on promotion of their own expertise. The broader the scope of services offered by an affiliated specialist hospital is, and the simpler and clearer the published menu of services for referring veterinarians is, the greater the opportunity for internal referrals will be.

- *Financing.* Financial constraints should be explicitly stated. The breadth of the mission and vision is determined by the amount of unfunded and underfunded work the affiliated group is willing to undertake, and it is wise to set that amount annually during the program-based budgeting process.

When the board extends the mission focus to the vision, their thoughts often become broader, more emotional, and more morally based; this generally makes the vision more difficult to achieve than the mission. Both mission focus and vision setting are essential for any governance board, but the terminology often differs. Taken together with the core values of tough decision making, mission focus and vision express not only what the organization is committed to do (here called the mission), but what it intends to do over longer periods of time (here called the vision). The vision should make clear what the organization hopes to achieve, what constraints it recognizes, and how it will do business. It typically includes

- How the organization should be viewed by both members and outsiders.

- The organizational philosophy that guides operational activities.

- The organization's concept of its strengths and weaknesses.

- The evaluation of community opportunities and strengths.

The core values, mission focus, and vision become the cornerstones for judging competing opportunities identified by strategic assessment of the environment. The best planning scenarios are actually several scenarios, developed by multiple board actions and members, involving technical and professional questions rather than policy issues. Initial scenarios should be abstract and ambiguous; they are made specific only after the alternatives and potential strategic opportunities have been evaluated. Strategic opportunities may include quantum shifts in service capabilities or market share, often by mergers and additional affiliations, and sometimes by outright acquisitions or joint ventures. Strategic opportunities require careful evaluation, since very large-scale capital investments are required. Once strategies and priorities are set, the planning effort largely leaves the board level. Delegation to daily operational levels is important to empower the staff to accept the mission, see the vision, and apply the core values.

In established boards, we routinely see a variation between what is written and what is done. The bylaws may clarify who bears the ultimate responsibility. Culturally and historically, however, the board may not have behaved that way, so when it comes time for the governance board to exercise its ultimate authority, it meets internal resistance from members within the system who say, "You can't make that decision without checking with us." The governance board quotes the bylaws, and the rebels within the system say, "Yeah, it is in the bylaws but we don't care what is in the bylaws, you've never done this before, so you can't do it now." And the system grinds to a halt.

We have seen practices with just two owners taking 60–120 days to make a decision simply because they fear failure. Anytime there is ambiguity in role and responsibility, there is a lack of strategic alignment; this causes an inability to execute strategic responses, and great opportunities are lost. When a governance board has a bylaw requirement but abdicates to the historical or cultural vestige of consensus-based decision making, the system strategy grinds the progress effort to a halt. A walk-the-talk process must be established concurrently with every board. Whenever we find two decision systems functioning concurrently, we have a disease that will eat away at the governance system. When there are too many historical variances, and a board must touch base with each entity before it can make a decision, then the governance board is dead. A dead board must be cremated and buried, and governance restructuring is required immediately.

Another failure to walk the talk occurs with governance conflict. Governance conflict exists when board task forces or committees, within a governance system, are continually fighting with each other. We have all seen this with professional associations and the traditional committee form of reference; who is funded and who is most important. A governance board can have the worst of both worlds, where gridlock and conflict exist simultaneously. Since both are inappropriate, there must be a way of changing them. We use some basic principles for system governance (these are our biases) in veterinary medicine affiliations:

- Get some form of community involvement in the governance structure, whether it be from the local VMA, a humane society, or even an animal owner. It is not unusual to find a corporate attorney or banker as an advisor to the board, and some even get voting privileges if they are animal owners.

- The staff spends a lot of time and energy for the practices involved; they have a right to examine policy decisions (the "why"). The position, "This is a community-based system; governance acts on the behalf of the community, because that is what a board is supposed to do, so we are the responsible stewards of our resources on behalf of the community," is not unusual. The board, through the executive team, must ensure that the staff understands the why of the decisions that are implemented.

- Is it more important that you have community members on your board, or is it more important that you have people on your board that have the skills that are necessary to make the meaningful governance decisions and lead the organization? If you can have both, marvelous!

- The board must be aware of the functional distinction of the players. If there is a radiologist, the expectation of image interpretation is a given, but the extension of prognosis and treatment is not. Board-certified emergency and critical care specialists have both internal medicine and surgery capabilities, but may not be credentialed by the board to perform all procedures if there are other specialists on staff available with greater skills and experience. If there are ultrasound capabilities, internal medicine could be credentialed for some procedures, and radiology for others, but the client (referring practice) must have the right to refer to the specialist of choice without internal paradigms being invoked.

- The specialty group hospitals have a potential for economy-of-scale savings in personnel management, centralized pharmacy, joint use wards and runs, central information technology (common computer system), and central medical supply, as well as internal referrals to other specialists. The governance board has the accountability for integration oversight, and any nonparticipant in the facility risks being decredentialed if he/she adversely affects the whole.

- A board can make any structural model work, if it selects heir options based on some conscious, predefined, explicit criteria to advance a specific system purpose. As a consulting team, we can make any rational governance system work, but the problem we have found is that many systems mix and match their decision process criteria so frequently that there is no one system to support. Consistency in mission focus, vision, and core values and reinforcement for major decisions are criteria for success.

- When we work as consultants to governance systems, it is our job to make sure that there is strategic alignment among all pieces of the system. It is the board's job to govern the organization; it is the centralized authority. As consultants we offer advice and an outside perspective, but we highly recommend decentralized decision making for daily operational activities. This is a very important concept, and if you disagree, fine, but you had better have some governing principle that precludes developing frustration within staff members who perceive this micromanagement as distrust and decision inactivity.

- We believe that any governance board must be able to make quick decisions and then task the executive team for their immediate implementation. If your board disagrees with this and selects the operational principle that consensus-based leadership, where everyone has authority, is better, the board won't be able to make quick decisions, and community-based strategic responses will not generally be possible. This board will usually take 120–180 days to make a decision.

- We believe very strongly that unless you have a very compelling reason not to do it, the philosophies and designs for management, clinical services, and governance should be similar. It makes no sense to have centralized management and decentralized governance. Yet, in practice, that is the choice many operations committees have made, by continually referring back to the shareholders for consensus. Some group practices and veterinary referral hospitals have streamlined management by centralizing the day-to-day operations, but have decentralized governance. Some non-healthcare businesses have opted for centralized governance and decentralized management, but as students of leadership trends, we don't believe anyone can make an argument for centralized management and decentralized governance.

- With affiliations, many practices choose to streamline (centralize) the operational facility management, then look at consolidating clinical relationships, without ever addressing the governance structure. How can a governance group lead if they are always dragging behind? It drives me crazy to see a board composed entirely of veterinarians, just because they are clinical experts. These specialists know how to deliver care, and they may know how to govern a closely held private practice, but they seldom know anything about strategic assessment of community demographics or environmental influences on organization behavior. Veterinarians are seldom recruited because of their big-business strategy or outreach capabilities. We must be willing to change the models of board selection. We still believe in majority veterinarian membership on boards, and with tough boundary decisions, it becomes critical. But we recommend focused doctor membership. What do we mean by this? We choose people to serve on boards, not just because they are veterinarians, but also because they have the skills that are necessary to pursue the board's mission, goals, and objectives.

- The IRS has changed the board requirements in not-for-profit human healthcare situations. It used to be that a 501(c)3 board could not have more than 20 percent primary providers on a healthcare board. Now there can be 49 percent interested parties (attending physicians, CEOs, employed staff, etc.) on the board. There have been no IRS rulings on veterinary medicine governance boards to date. On most hospital boards, the chief of professional staff (CPS) serves as an ex-officio member of the governance board; if there is a veterinary hospital CPS, this should be considered, because this individual is supposed to be the liaison between the governance board and the professional staff.

- We like to reserve certain powers within the governance board and develop the parameters to give the board the authority to act decisively. One of the powers we like to reserve to the board is the so-called nuclear button. If a board member doesn't measure up, he/she can be removed at will. When the board has this power, and a member of the board starts to veer away from the core values, vision, or mission focus, the board must have a mechanism to immediately correct the situation. The board can say, "Please come back," but if the aberrant member says, "No, the board is wrong, we are moving in a direction that is bad for my part of this organization," the governance board must have the ability to remove him/her. However, when a board continually removes members, it is time to nuke the system, that is, to release everyone and reconstitute the board in order to refocus the board on the core business.

Making It Happen for You

Management in transition means managers in transition; change is the rule! The new look means the old habits must be reassessed in light of the new core values. Hospital boards are increasingly facing the challenge of integrating polarity rather than making black or white decisions, and one of the great challenges of the administrator is balancing these polarities with daily operational needs. We are seeing affiliated hospital environments getting into other types of businesses as well, including boarding, grooming, physical therapy, alternative medicine, hosting specialists, and internal referrals, just to name a few. Any type of board should be able to accept this expansion role, but boards need to continuously monitor and improve themselves.

Boards must assess how they spend their time, how they can modify their structure, what instruction the new members receive, whether there is strategic alignment among the pieces of the system, and similar boundary issues. This all becomes a very important challenge for the board, and a greater challenge for the administrator. The board must lead the system, and it must lead on the basis of where the system is going, not where the system has been. The executive team, led by the hospital administrator, is the real key to effective governance. If we look at a typical board, we find there are very few things it can actually control. If it doesn't control these few, the board will not be efficient or effective.

Setting the Agenda

For effective board functioning, the administrator must orchestrate these board activities:

- The time the board spends together.

- The board's utilization of time.

Its time together is the single most precious commodity the board has, and that is one of the things that makes a board absolutely fascinating. A board does not legally exist unless it is meeting: the only time a board exists is between raps of the gavel. Individual board members have no authority whatsoever. One of the best ways of controlling a board's time is by controlling its agenda. Most boards we work with do not control their agendas. Amazingly, when we ask the board of an emergency hospital or specialty referral center who controls the agenda, or even who sets the agenda, most board members do not know the process by which their own agenda is set. Agendas rule time utilization. This is why an annual list of tough issues must be developed, and why a tough issue leads each meeting agenda. Core values and mission focus must be clear, so the two or three hours a month the board has together can be used to set policy, make decisions, and better define boundaries. Consider the following:

- A consulting test we do with established boards, and I suggest you do this, is to pull out the agenda for today and two from previous meetings a year or two ago, white out the dates so they are unreadable, mix them up, and pass them out to the board. The question we ask is, "Can you tell which agenda is for today's meeting?" About 60 percent of the time the agendas are identical.

- If you have an agenda for a meeting for today and an agenda from two years ago that look the same, that means you are dealing with the same issues you were dealing with two years ago.

- The agendas of good boards change. They change almost from meeting to meeting as different issues ascend or descend in level of importance, consistent with the identified strategic plan. Good boards control the agenda.

- Many boards put everything into a constant agenda (the same outline every time): the approval of the minutes, the receipt of the profit and loss statement from the CPA, and decisions that boards are legally required to make but aren't that important in the big picture. Constant agendas place all issues on the same level, making it difficult to apportion time to critical issues that require discussion. Use of constant agendas is therefore a detriment to progress.

- Most boards will take the most meaningless, boring, censorious nonsense and put it first on their agenda. As the administrator, you can lump these items together into one agenda item, send out the information to the board members ahead of the meeting date, and say, "Read this—if there are no questions, we are done." This procedure makes more time for the important issues.

- The average board saves the most important critical issues for last, and they often don't appear on the agenda except as new business. We are very simple people so we have very simple suggestions: (1) identify what the most important critical issues are (and many boards have not done that), and (2) put them first on the agenda.

Board members at any level must understand which issues it is most important to spend their time on. To do this, the board needs to review the system's vision on those issues. Furthermore, board members must have the discipline to put blinders on and not discuss issues which are seductive, which they would simply like to get into, which are situational, and which are not on-track with the strategy of the organization.

When a veterinary hospital administrator works with his/her board, he/she needs to keep two questions foremost: What is the mission? What is the plan? In seeking an answer to the second question, the administrator should ask what the three or four most critical important issues confronting the organization or system in the next couple of years will be. Most boards can't tell you. They don't know what the critical issues are, so they have no way of organizing their direction or their time to address those issues. Once the administrator has identified what the critical issues are and put them at the top of the agenda, the board can deal with the most critical issues, and the executive team has direction.

Providing Relevant Information

When the administrator has structured the agenda, the executive team can then structure the information. Many practices are struggling to create good management information systems, but they forget to create good governance information systems. Board reports are not warmed-over management information. Don't send the board management reports, committee minutes, or even written task force progress reports. Boards should get information that is relevant to the critical issues in a format that is relevant to the function of the board; such information should include items that are big picture, community trend oriented, and future directed.

- The 20 or 30 percent of meeting time that the board gets to monitor the system should be in the framework of graphic indicators, charts that show the indicators and the upper and lower control limits. Board members don't have to be financial geniuses; the finance task force, with advice, should develop no more than 12 financial indicators, with upper and lower control limits. When board members see the indicators are within the control limits, they don't need to spend any time on them.

- When the indicators begin approaching the control limits, questions should be expected; footnotes can offer the explanations. That is how an administrator can get monitoring the past down to 20–30 percent of a board's time. When an administrator gives the board members graphical indicator information in advance, it enables the board to begin planning and creating the future.

Choosing a Daily Operational Structure

After board meetings have been orchestrated for maximum productivity, the administrator gets to the issue of choosing the best operational structure, which is critical for daily operations. Look at the major areas of administrative implementation for a key to establishing the correct structure:

- Centralized human resource management

- Information system operations (central computer)

- Central medical supply (CMS) and distribution systems

- Drug inventory management

- Accounts receivable support

- Accounts payable and internal billing systems

- Committees or task forces from the services (optional)

As the administrator, you must understand both the why and how of the operational structures needed to support the board's strategy. Go back to Winston Churchill's comment, "First we create our structures, then they create us." If the administrator does not control the operational structures, the executive team will become their prisoners. The linchpin of effective leadership in a governance board-based system is founded on one question: Once the board makes meaningful decisions and sets robust policies, how does the administrator make it happen? If the administrator does not control time (sequencing of events), the board's tough-issue agenda, the graphic information presented to the board, and the daily operational structures, then it will be very difficult to implement those meaningful decisions and robust policies. Here are three quick thoughts about the implementation process:

- Our bias is toward streamlining operations, but you can make any structure work. The secret is clear expectations, with crystal clear boundaries, which can be met at least 60 percent of the time. Pride in performance comes when expectations are exceeded, and staff pride is perceived as quality by clients.

- Here is a very good diagnostic tool for innovation, and it is also indicative of the operational process. What percent of staff suggestions gets implementation within 48 hours? If your answer is "less than 60 percent," you have an executive challenge. Veterinary hospital administrators working with a governance board need the latitude to make operational decisions, including setting significant unilateral spending limits.

- There must be authority vested in the hospital administrator to mediate boundary disputes by facilitated discussion of the involved parties. If the administrator concludes that (1) there is a problem situation and (2) it needs to change, there must be a way for addressing the problem at the operational level. If the administrator can facilitate changing environmental distractions, then resolution is possible. If not, resolution will not occur, and the board will need to become involved. When the board becomes overloaded with such process interventions, the result is poor strategic response to opportunities and a dysfunctional relationship with the executive team.

Minimizing Friction

The final concern for the hospital administrator working within a board-centered governance system is how to minimize the difficulties and risks associated with board relationships. Obviously, this is a complex matter with many personality and environmental variables, but there are five guidelines for improving the effectiveness and prolonging the tenure of hospital administrators.

Hire the Right Person for the Job

The old habit of promoting from within will seldom work in an affiliated practice facility for two reasons: allegiance and breadth of mission experience/knowledge. There are many facets of organizational behavior, economics, facility planning, logistics, human resources, strategic planning, and related skills that the average veterinary practice does not develop in its managers. The Certified Veterinary Practice Manager designation (from the Veterinary Hospital Managers Association) is one skill set, as is the Master in Healthcare Administration degree. A diplomate of the American College of Healthcare Administrators has passed boards (there is a 60-plus percent fail rate), oral and written, to be certified in the skill set needed for this task. These people do not come cheap and can start at a salary almost double that of the average practice manager; but they are worth it.

Make Actions, Procedures, and Assignments of
Responsibility Consistent

Actions, procedures, and assignments of responsibility should be consistent. The governance structure involves a group of individuals that relates frequently to dozens of others. Written records, formal procedures, and adherence to a consistent set of expectations are necessary for the group members to work effectively together. The by-laws of the board should specify the foundation procedures, and well-run hospitals adhere to their by-laws in order to gain predictability. Many people become inpatient with such a formality, and a hospital can establish a deliberate tradition of informality, but only within certain formal constraints.

Agree on Short-term Goals and Expectations

The board and hospital administrator should agree on short-term (usually one-year) goals and expectations and should review progress toward them on a quarterly basis. The expectations for the hospital administrator are generally more ambiguous than those for others on the executive team, and they are more subject to unexpected outside influences. On occasion, the administrator's goals and objectives must be radically revised in mid-course; flexibility is therefore required of the board and the administrator. Expectations for the veterinary hospital administrator must be related to the goals of the institution as a whole. The administrator's charter emerges from other activities of the governing board, particularly the long-range plan and the approved, annual, program-based budget.

Make the Employment Contract Clear

The board and the hospital administrator should have a mutual understanding of the administrator's employment contract. There is always a contract, and the formality of the contract depends on the situation, but more detailed contracts have become popular in recent years for this position. The contract should specify any departures from the usual duties expected, mechanisms for review of performance and compensation, and procedures for amendment and revision of the operational charter. It should also state procedures for termination of the relationship, including appropriate protection for both the hospital and the administrator. Properly performed, the hospital administrator's job in an affiliated practice facility is, and always has been, a high-risk endeavor. Thus, even handshake agreements should include appropriate protections for both parties in the event the administrator leaves the institution.

Establish Fair Compensation

Compensation should be based on market conditions and should contain incentives for effective performance. In general, the only fair and reasonable guidelines for designing a compensation package, in the marketplace, are what the institution would have to pay a similarly prepared individual, and what the person could earn in similar employment elsewhere. The high visibility of the hospital administrator, internally and externally, and the relatively high income of the position compared to general practice situations, often tempt unsophisticated board members to use other criteria (which will cause difficulty and conflict for the board). The value and contributions of a skilled veterinary hospital administrator is almost impossible to determine; comparisons to other personnel are therefore problematic. No matter how much other people earn, if a similar position would pay more elsewhere, the administrator is underpaid. On the other hand, if the administrator's compensation package is above the marketplace, the hospital's money is being wasted. The marketplace used to determine pay should be the same one used in the selection procedure. In this emerging field of veterinary hospital administration, the market for people trained and experienced in effective affiliated practice environments is national. When determining compensations, consider the following:

- *Compensation* includes payments in addition to salary that often are unique to the hospital administrator. Besides salary, the package can contain benefits offered to all staff, special benefits offered to selected key persons, bonuses and merit increases, disposition of incidental income earned by the administrator, and an agreement on both voluntary and involuntary termination compensation.

- *Special benefits* usually exploit the mutual interests of the hospital, the administrator, and the income tax laws. These can include payments for housing, transportation, education, association dues, registration and certification fees, and deferred income provisions.

- *Bonuses and achievement incentives* are more common in established practice environments, based on excess earnings or savings (when compared to the annual program-based budget).

- *Annual reviews and merit increases* are expected, separate from the performance planning process with the board. In the review, the hospital administrator is rewarded for his or her efforts toward the agreed upon goals. The amount of the merit increase is determined by the board, which considers the overall success of the institution and the contributions to the development of the executive team.

Administrator Skills and Performance Factors

To accomplish everything discussed in the previous pages, the veterinary hospital administrator must bring a very special skill set to bear on the operations of the facility. This set includes technical, leadership, decision-making, and character-based skills. *Technical skills* are acquired through formal education and experience and include image marketing, investment management, construction planning, human resource management, and client solicitation. *Leadership skills* are developed almost exclusively through experience, and they are based on strong human relation skills, but they are difficult to test, so review of experiences and checking references are essential in the screening process. *Decision-making skills* are concerned with quality as well as quantity, and the style of leadership, from autocratic to democratic, should vary with the situation (e.g., an exclusively autocratic style tears at the fabric of cooperation and caring healthcare delivery, but may be required in times of major crisis). *Character-based skill sets* include ethics, emotional strength, commitment, and bioethical compassion. Administrators are in high-stress situations every day, and they must have an internal mind-set that pushes them to care and nurture others regardless of their own work pressures. It is probably true that character can be strengthened, and the ability to handle stress can be learned, but these skills are all based on a balanced life. The American College of Healthcare Executives **requires** its diplomates to stay involved in community activities, and failure to stay actively involved is cause for loss of certification (and diplomate boards are required at five-year intervals, so there is a true check and balance system involved).

Measures of the hospital administrator's performance can take many forms, but there are some basic objective measures that should always be addressed:

- *Demand and market share measures.* Administrators can influence demand by effective planning, operations, service relationships, and promotion. Market share is a relative demand, as opposed to absolute demand, and is an internal progression measure.

- *Outcome measures.* These can include informal satisfaction surveys, quality of output, technical performance, staff recruitment and retention, and stratified random samples of the community perceptions (often done by focus groups of referring veterinarians).

- *Resource consumption (cost and efficacy) measures.* Cost measures are readily available from annual budgets and monthly reports, as income can be, but for the board, it needs to presented as a readily available aggregate, such as cost per discharge, income per FTE staff member, and other ratios that reflect meaningful input-output relationships.

- *Profit and financial condition measures.* Expectations for profit arise from the program-based budgeting process, and the programs, while out of the hands of the administrator, can be tracked by the executive team and fine-tuned by administrator negotiations with participating specialty services. The success of the individual participants means success for the facility.

- *Subjective assessment (process evidence supporting outcomes).* Outside influences are a diverse set of exceptions and demands and may be reflected in the recruitment programs for staff and referring practices, as well as in in-service training programs and staff development efforts. The staff deserves respect, responsibility, and recognition; their perception of these three Rs are subjective yet essential for their pride and subsequent facility success.

- *Prior board agreements.* Obligations to support the hospital, board reports, information technology, community relations, planning, and forensic/legal concerns can affect this management by objective measurement. But these factors must be kept in equitable balance with the other measurements (some inexperienced administrators prefer to do tasking, which means they are not bold and robust in the decision-making process).

- *Nonquantifiable achievements.* Recognition from the community, involvement in civic clubs, and other activities that bring awareness of the facility and administrator are icing on the cake in most cases, but they concurrently increase the institutional awareness of community needs and demands, thereby assisting the strategic response capability of the board.

- *Executive team development and harmony.* Self-evaluation is always expected, and this is often confused with specific reports or achievements, but the organizational climate is a critical factor that must be evaluated when assessing the effectiveness of any veterinary hospital administrator. A true administrator will develop people through work, while the traditional manager gets work done through people.

Governance for the twenty-first century and engineering veterinary boards for a new era in veterinary healthcare delivery require a partnership of strategic planning and operational excellence; the veterinary hospital administrator ensures the partnership functions well on a continuing basis. The hospital administrators in well-run veterinary facilities appear deceptively passive. They let the external world and individual members build motivation and devote their attention to developing and promoting the environmental factors that affect the facility as a whole. Critical attention is paid by the hospital administrator to the communication of differing viewpoints, timely management of the decision structure, consistent application of the mission focus and core values, and pursuit of the facility vision.

WHEN IS IT TIME FOR GOVERNANCE?

The following statements should be applied to the veterinary organization in question, with "as it is now" answers, rather than "what we hope we can make it" desires of the current practice culture. The survey applies to multi-owner entities, but the principles belong to any leader, so anyone may use it for self-assessment.

Yes	Maybe	No	Critical Operational Objective
___	___	___	Known core values—inviolate beliefs that all can depend on.
___	___	___	Core values based on the beliefs of the practice leadership.
___	___	___	There is a shared (with the staff) mission focus, and it must be believed.
___	___	___	Mission focus is used to help make difficult decisions.
___	___	___	There is shared confidence in each other's behavior.
___	___	___	Nonquantifiable achievements are recognized at least monthly.
___	___	___	Operational expectations are stated as outcome measures.
___	___	___	Information is made relational for decision-making purposes.
___	___	___	The big picture view is required **before** operation philosophy changes.
___	___	___	Monthly staff meetings are minimized.
___	___	___	Meeting agendas are required—there is always a problem to solve.
___	___	___	Unscheduled issues at meetings are tabled until the next meeting.
___	___	___	Program/procedure adjustments are made at least quarterly.
___	___	___	Resource consumption (cost and efficacy) measures are used.
___	___	___	Profit and financial condition measures are reviewed quarterly.
___	___	___	Subjective assessments are used for recognitions (process evidence-supporting outcomes).
___	___	___	Program-based decisions require expense centers and income centers to be matched business entities.
___	___	___	Isolated-perspective, expense-based decisions are minimized.
___	___	___	Reinvestment in the future is a fiscal commitment to action.
___	___	___	Prevention of bad data is a quarterly adjustment process.
___	___	___	Prior operating agreements are reviewed at least annually.
___	___	___	There is no killing of the cash cow without replacement stock.
___	___	___	Strategic response is community-centered, not practice-centered.
___	___	___	Demand and market share measures exist.
___	___	___	There is no protection of the cash cow if it has outlived its usefulness.

Yes	Maybe	No	Critical Operational Objective
―	―	―	Commitment to the practice entity is a condition of leadership.
―	―	―	Dedication and loyalty by individuals are recognized in public.
―	―	―	There are methods to deal with those resisting change rather than leading it.
―	―	―	Attention to process does not mean control of operations.
―	―	―	People can be and **must** be removed quickly for cause.
―	―	―	Adverse counseling is done in private.
―	―	―	Management for stability and status quo is accepted as bad.
―	―	―	Leadership accepts change revolution as a standard need.
―	―	―	Job description for decision makers exist.
―	―	―	Methods and criteria for management reorganization exist.
―	―	―	Doctors do not conflict either in public or in front of staff.
―	―	―	Middle managers do not cut down leadership.
―	―	―	Executive team development and harmony exist.
―	―	―	Conflicts of interest are never permitted.
―	―	―	No independent veto authority is held by any team member.
―	―	―	Leadership is centered not in details but in outcomes.
―	―	―	Strategic assessment has replaced operational guidance.
―	―	―	This is a fun place to work—it's a pleasure to come in each day.

SCORING THE GOVERNANCE SURVEY

All "Yes"—This is atypical, likely biased, and should be retaken by consensus.

All "No"—This is atypical, likely biased, and should be retaken by consensus.

"Yes" answers are in the minority (<22)—This is a practice where organizational realignment is indicated immediately, and an independent governance structure is likely indicated. You have already proven you can't do it with what you have as resources and experience, and you need a strong veterinary governance consultant to assist you. Sorry about that.

"Yes" answers between 22 and 34—You are doing some things right, but you need to develop a more predictable approach to the practice. A consulting team or practice team seminar may be needed to tailor the current literature to your specific veterinary practice and get the healthcare delivery system stabilized. At the end of 90 days, after enacting the changes suggested by the consulting team or practice seminar, assess improvements. If your score is still under 34, immediate organizational realignment is indicated so that you do not lose the momentum of your initial effort. You were not able to turn the corner with the internal resources and experience cycle available. You need a strong veterinary governance consultant to assist you in establishing an independent governance structure.

"Yes" answers between 34 and 43—This is like getting a "B" in "sandbox" at kindergarten. A client-centered team effort is needed to develop a greater sense of healthcare delivery effectiveness. You may also require a consulting team to assist your management and leadership team(s) in developing an implementation and transition plan for tailoring the principles and procedures in the current literature to your specific practice needs. There are good leadership and learning organization texts available; allowing the staff to develop to their full potential as veterinary extenders is building the learning organization! If you can slowly improve your score over time, a governance structure may not be required at this point in time.

Turf wars—Regardless of the survey score(s), if there is any intraoperational debate over client access or scope of services by specific providers, a central hospital with off-site owners, a multi-specialty practice, a shareholder-supervised emergency practice, or any other form of turf war, a new governance structure is required. You must seek outside, credentialed expertise to mediate: you cannot be a prophet in your own town. Consider establishing a consulting engagement with a strong veterinary governance consultant, to assist you in establishing an independent governance structure that meets your operational needs.

3 Expansion in the New Millennium—Representing the Group

When faced with two evils, I prefer to try the one I have never experienced; it is more fun!
—Mae West

In the expanding practice, representing the group is one of the most challenging leadership skills, for the leadership and management staff alike. It is most often described as a dual-role position, one representing the practice philosophy to all others, and one representing the clients and staff back to the practice leadership. Sorry to say, with the mergers and affiliations we are beginning to see in veterinary medicine, it will become more difficult in the new millennium.

The Return to Core Values

The revised management expectations in the new American veterinary practice will require the uncommon leader to build a team who can make the strategic responses required to grab opportunity as it races by the front door of the practice. The team must be able to bond clients at every contact, which means the leadership must first bond the staff to the practice. The day of disposable staff is over; you must treat staff as you want your clients to be treated. The team must also work and play well with other community organizations, including other veterinary practices. In this era of e-mail and immediate electronic communications, there is no longer the luxury of slow response or incremental decisions. The strategic planning that required a systematic assessment of the next three to five years and an incremental plan for adjusting and adapting to the changing environment is no longer the route to success in veterinary practice. Successful practices of the future will be learning organizations.

To build a learning organization, one must address the issue of how to survive in a profession that is doubling in knowledge every 24 months. In-service training is one tool for implementing the continuous quality improvement that is a hallmark of the learning organization, and relying on the brains of every member of the team is another. In the management transition of the future, each veterinary practice team leader will have to provide fuel for the innovation engine. The challenge will be determining who the team members are representing and why the practice needs to start the change process (it is no longer an issue of change or not, but rather an issue of why change is needed and how fast it should come).

To establish an accurate practice direction, the practice leadership needs core values. In representing the group, and in a diversified demand relationship, everyone in the practice must know and embrace the core values of the practice. Core values are central to the practice, so everyone in the practice must understand that

- Core values must be inviolate.

- When strategic response decisions are made, they must support the core values and the core business of the practice.

- The days of doctor-driven exceptions will be over; staff members deserve a high level of consistency, predictability, and dependability from the leadership.

- The operational and behavioral boundaries inherent within the core values must be discussed and understood by all.

- Outcome definitions will replace process controls, and the staff will use core values to adjust the systems for continuous quality improvement.

- The outcome expectations associated with the implementation of core value decisions must be known at the outset, since exceeding expectations drives future staff participation.

- When staff members have respect and responsibility and are given recognition for exceeding expectations, they will show pride in performance.

- The clients accessing the practice will perceive staff pride as quality and will pay premium prices for the feeling of confidence, or peace of mind, that is associated with that feeling.

Managing Multiple Practices

The management of multiple practices was a rare art in the 1980s but has become more common in the 1990s; in the twenty-first century, it will be a mandate for economies of scale and profitability. The decision to open another practice weighs on the minds of many practitioners today; in our consulting practice, about one in five practices visited asks about the advisability of this type of expansion. Some practices want to increase their exposure or their availability to a larger segment of the population, while others want to prevent other practices from infringing on their territory. Some realize that they need more inpatients, so they open outpatient facilities within reasonable commuting distance for better self-referrals. The reasons for opening additional practices are many, but the challenges in management remain similar.

The economy-of-scale challenge facing many practices today is the decision to diversify, internally or externally. In the process of external diversification, the decision to diversify becomes more difficult when we look at multiple practices, especially if a consistency of patient care is desired. There are key challenges and alternatives that must be addressed to assist the diversification transition. Paraprofessionals and professionals destined for another facility should be empowered and required to practice new middle management skills at the parent practice level; requiring employees to learn new management skills during on-the-job training, often called trial by fire, is a worst-case scenario, and should be avoided. Consider the following:

- In a multifacility practice, the owner/director must practice the skills of delegation, empowerment, and sharing leadership so that each person's behavior on the management/leadership team becomes predictable.

- In a multiowner group of practices, the group administrator or contract manager represents the joint philosophy of the owners and must practice the skills of delegation, empowerment, and sharing leadership so that each person's behavior on the management/leadership team becomes predictable.

- Each veterinary facility, regardless of ownership and operational structure, must have someone responsible on site to answer that urgent question, whether it be on health care, staff relations, or procurement actions.

- In a shared facility with multiple practices (e.g., a specialty hospital) or a facility with shared ownership (e.g., emergency practice shareholders), the administrator may have a single physical structure but multiple sets of demands. These demands are usually best resolved with the implementation of the governance concepts discussed in Chapter Two.

Leadership Essentials

The Premise

Managing multiple practices is no different than executive management of a single large facility; you get things done by developing others to a level of performance that can be trusted. The challenge here is that very few veterinarians manage their practices through others; *control* is usually their watchword. This situation has not allowed the average practice manager to have a mentor who can develop his/her skills as a leader. The average veterinarian is usually a conservative, independent, I-can-do-it-better healthcare professional; executive management (organizing and controlling through other managers) is not his/her forte.

The Veterinary Hospital Managers Association (VHMA @ 518-433-8911) has long discussed the contract manager, someone who serves many practices in one area. In simplest economic terms, one well-trained, veterinary-savvy, administrative leader can mentor six to nine on-site, single-practice managers; can centralize the human resource management and inventory procurement (economy-of-scale factor); and can be a trainer of trainers for the practices supported. This means that if each single practice pays this highly skilled administrative leader $1,000 per month for one half-day a week on site, plus telephone support as needed, and there are six practices involved, the administrator earns $6,000 per month ($72,000 per year). It also means either half-day on-site practice support six days a week, or three full days of on-site practice support, with a drive between facilities over the lunch hour.

The certified veterinary practice manager (CVPM) designation by VHMA and the diplomate designation by ACHE indicate that the designated person knows the answers and understands the healthcare profession; they do indicate how effectively that person can share his/her skills. As with any professional (CVPMs and ACHE diplomates, are both professionals in healthcare administration, one is just a bit more specialized than the other), skills and knowledge are the tip of the iceberg; it is the attitude below the waterline that makes the relationship work. These professionals are mini-consultants, and any good consultant must start as a chameleon, developing the programs around the practice's core values, mission focus, staff strengths, and community market niche (if it has been identified). A great group administrator (what I prefer to call the contract manager of VHMA), with six different practices as regular clients, will likely have seven to 10 different management approaches going simultaneously.

New leadership skills must be learned and implemented on a recurring basis by anyone who wishes to be a reputable group administrator. These skills include the following:

- Team building.
  - ✓ Knowing and using the resources of the group.
  - ✓ Understanding the characteristics and needs of the group members.
  - ✓ Using effective communication (getting **and** giving meaningful information).

- Developing trust and sharing leadership.
  - ✓ Program and operational planning (value-based).
  - ✓ Delegation and individual empowerment (outcome orientation).
  - ✓ Evaluation, coaching, and counseling (clear expectations).
  - ✓ Effective teaching (from discovery to competency review).

- Developing the middle managers.
  - ✓ Practicing situational leadership (cannot be all things for all people).
  - ✓ Fostering group development (understanding the dynamics of change).
  - ✓ Fostering personal relationships (establish "barrier busting" paradigms).
  - ✓ Giving internal practice promotions (we only sell "peace of mind").

- Exhibiting personal executive leadership skills.
  - ✓ Setting the example (actions speaking louder than words).
  - ✓ Practicing continuous quality improvement (every day in every way).

Training Requirements

Multiple practices require sharing leadership, delegating both authority and responsibility for action, and trusting others to maintain the core values and mission focus of the practice. Because they are unique, each practice in the stable of the group administrator may require a different operational perspective. In the new multiple practice environment, owners will require specialized leadership training before the training of the staff can begin: there must be consensus at the top before there is implementation at the bottom. For the new administrator looking to branch out, the multiple practice environment will require learning new leadership skill habits that will need to be perfected at the original facility before he/she attempts to train others and export the programs to other facilities. A good group administrator will

- Have a technical skill set above the community average

- Demonstrate a noteworthy leadership skill set at all times

- Give credit and take blame when working with others

- Catch people doing things right and praise frequently in public

- Consider mistakes a learning effort and counsel always in private

- Always tell the truth with compassion and never use brutal honesty

- Disagree with issues but never make someone else "wrong"

- Develop other people through work and hear their caring intentions

- Be available as promised and predictable in delivery

- Do the right things, for the right reason, at the right time

Performance Measurement

Without a yardstick, there is no measurement. Without measurement, there is no control. Without control, there is no business expectation for the practice. Without a business expectation for the practice, there is no way to measure practice business excellence.
—Dr. T.E. Catanzaro

Accountability

Accountability is more than just responsibility. It is setting clear measurement expectations that are within the control of those who have the related responsibility. The person who is given responsibility for outcome expectations must also be given the related accountability and authority. That person needs to know that he/she "owns" that segment of the practice success goal(s). However, to set success goals for something, you must first be able to measure it, and measurement requires appropriate data.

The ability to capture relevant practice management data must be established before a program-based cash budget is implemented. Each practice has its own operational profile, but there can be common indicators of performance. These indicators must be understood and accepted not only by the management team, but also by the CPA, the banker, and the lawyer advising the diversification. This means clearly determining and defining the key financial and administrative indicators that should be used as diagnostic indicators.

Diagnostic indicators are interwoven with goals and objectives for both veterinary healthcare standards and profit-based relationships. These management indicators must be limited to less than 30 factors (management focus must be healthcare directed, not reporting directed) and must be measurable and easily tracked. Examples of indicators include, but are not limited to

- Healthcare service (procedures) goals

- Gross income per month

- Changes in gross income from previous month and previous year

- Net income per month

- Doctor-hours per transaction

- Staff-hours per transaction

- Percent gross for paraprofessional salaries

- New client rates (and referral rates from happy clients)

- Average client transaction (ACT) trend

- Diagnostic ratio (diagnostic and pharmacy sales, by individual doctor)

- Cost of goods sold (nutrition separate, large and small animal separate, etc.)

- Similar action, expense, and income factors

Reporting

The need to establish expectations for feedback and summary of the management indicators is critical to managing multiple facilities. Accuracy and timeliness, as well as ease of use, must be considered when choosing a reporting system. In most veterinary practice situations, QuickBooks and QuickPay are the logical tools for the group administrator to use as a managerial accounting system. Regular reports and summaries of management indicators help on-site operators understand what elements are important to the ownership, what elements will be examined in reports, how the data will be presented, and what is needed to be seen as successful.

As staff needs to receive feedback from the ownership, the ownership needs to receive feedback from the staff. To this end, owners must develop critical leadership skill of staff meeting management. Frequent staff meetings (at least weekly for the entire team) keep practices working toward common goals. The ability to bring multiple management minds to bear on a specific challenge at one site is an important strength of a multiple-practice operation. While the ownership agenda will need to be published and distributed a few days prior to each meeting, the meetings themselves must be based on the ownership listening rather than talking. This is often achieved by rotating the meeting chairmanship among the attendees.

Performance Evaluation

Comparisons

The hardest management factor to master is usually objectivity. Everyone is a victim of his/her own experience; good group administrators have a broad vase of experience and realize that not all practices are similar. The values of the organization must be constant, but step-by-step goals and objectives need to be tailored to the competitive environment of the specific practice being addressed. Each facility must be compared to itself, not to other facilities. Data for each element being managed must be watched for progress in relation to similar data from that specific facility. For group administrators, the incremental improvement of a practice compared to itself is the yardstick of excellence, **never** the national averages. Always remember the Catanzaro definition of average: the best of the worst **or** the worst of the best. No veterinarian, and no healthcare staff member, wants to strive for either of the average classifications, so quit using the average as a yardstick.

Goals and objectives must be set based on the strengths of the individual facility and its staff. Staff members are different, and each facility must organize itself to capitalize on its specific human resource capabilities and on its catchment area demographics (also known as client profiles). The strength in multiple practices is capitalizing on the diversity of demand. A complex could have a central facility with specialists and multiple board-certified veterinarians, yet also operate a discount vaccination clinic for the lower income population; or a feline practice could be established that accesses the specialists without having to cater to canine or avian populations.

Analysis

The analysis of operations needs to be based on practice-specific expectations. A group administrator will have a set of yardsticks for each practice, as well as some internal controls that are standard expectations, including segregation of function, till close-out techniques, separation of petty cash and change funds, and other good management practices. The newly established program-based budget, the practice management indicators, and team harmony are integrated elements that must be concurrently evaluated. In new ventures, paralysis by analysis is a common problem. The multi-practice operator will never have all the information needed for an errorless decision. In fact, in the better managed human healthcare field, the success rate of new, great, diversification ideas is about 40 percent at maximum.

Operational analysis can be micro or macro in approach; an integrated combination of the two views is better than either approach separately. An internal control management example would be comparing the number of rabies vaccination charges to the sequential number of tags or certificates used and to the inventory use rate. The data for these comparisons should come from three different reports, so subordinate employees will not think of adjusting the figures to match expectations. While there are many methods available for analyzing data, the three critical issues are the benefit to the patient/client, the benefit to the staff, and the cost-benefit assessment.

Internal Controls

A Dozen Signal Flares

*Most cash loss is due to trusted employees; if you
didn't trust them, they wouldn't be handling the cash!*
—Dr. T.E. Catanzaro

Internal controls in most veterinary practices are as weak as the internal controls in any family setting. This is to be expected. Most veterinary staff are paid as if they were adolescents on an allowance; it isn't a retirement wage. Most people are hired onto the staff because they are nice people; they are trusted because that is the most common element in the veterinary practitioner's way of life. Veterinarians don't see their practice as a small business and do not approach the cash flow as if it needed to be controlled; they just want more cash flow.

As examples, we present four practices that have discovered staff theft, misappropriation, or other forms of embezzlement. Here are the facts as we know them:

- *Practice one.* This very busy one-man practice had no itemized receipts, and everything was "trusted." We established a super bill and a "one-write" receipt log. The trusted receptionist was found taking receipts home because she could no longer just skim cash.

- *Practice two.* This was a solid, two-veterinarian practice with a great receptionist who wrote personal checks, then cashed them from the cash drawer. When the checks were returned due to insufficient funds, she handled the case personally, for the bank and practice, thereby saving her from the review process. She remained undetected until the doctor started to look at the reconciliations.

- *Practice three.* This struggling two-veterinarian, small animal practice, after establishing a charting system, discovered they spent more money on pet food than they took in. Accountability for movement of the food was then assigned to the technicians, and **nothing** could leave the retail stock area without being logged onto a clipboard for later practice adjustment (to boarding costs or staff and doctor sale). The practice now operates in excess of 30 percent profit monthly.

- *Practice four.* This large, mixed animal practice has a computer system with no internal audit trail and very poor summary software; $40,000 was missing, and the loss was blamed on computer error.

As part of the consult, one of the veterinarians was assigned to start monitoring the cash flow system, including establishing a paired chart-of-accounts system, and he got the "loss" down to $10,000. The daily close-out system (with nightly bank deposits) was never fully implemented; everything was stuffed in a drawer and left until the morning for someone else to balance. Known cash overages did not appear on the deposits, thereby alerting owners to the skimming.

After an embezzlement, excuses routinely provided to the insurance company to account for the embezzlement include the following: (1) The doctor's lack of time and/or business experience. (2) The limited number of employees (which precluded the segregation of function). (3) Money was handled only by the receptionist team (but there was only one receptionist). (4) The lack of generally accepted accounting practices (GAAP). (5) And in most practices, the **failure** of the accountant (CPA) to be involved in the internal controls and the variance analysis of the practice's fiscal operations. Given these excuses and the potential most every practice has for lost cash, watch for these signal flares that indicate danger:

- The receptionist operates with an open cash drawer (no receipts).

- Receipts are made after the client departs, when there is "more time."

- The receptionist never takes a vacation and is very protective of her turf.

- The cash-handling person displays unexplained wealth (expensive vacations, new clothes, new jewelry, etc.).

- The petty cash fund (or worse, the change fund) has IOUs instead of receipts (personal checks are also a warning sign here).

- The money handler never asks for raises, takes a long time to cash paychecks, or never needs to leave early (during closeout) on days when she/he works alone.

- Invoices or records are rewritten (allegedly for neatness), often working overtime after everyone else has left.

- Accounting records are not up-to-date, or must be taken home by an employee to close out the period.

- Clients complain about errors in their statements, or about a lack of a statement following a procedure/service.

- Cash, as a percentage of total revenues, decreases each month, most often in direct relationship to the slowed practice growth.

- The billing person gives vague reasons for writing off uncollectible accounts (or client accounts require more adjustments for error than in the past).

- Staff members are not required to close out the change fund and balance against the daily receipts before departure (shortages and overages are accepted variances in daily activities).

Any of the above could exist in any practice. It could be a normal occurrence. On the other hand, the presence of one or more of these could be a warning, a signal flare of danger. If one or more are detected, a close and thorough review of your cash collection, billing, and product procurement and distribution systems is in order.

Trust Everybody, but Cut the Cards

Internal control is based on segregation of function, or the inability of any one person to have control of all the steps in a process. For instance, when someone orders supplies, a different person receives the items, checks off the shipping documents as received, and gives the annotated documents to the doctor for transmittal to the person who pays the bills. In cases where there is a computer, every client should be logged through the appointment log (even walk-ins), assigned a circle sheet (travel sheet) for the visit (even over-the-counter sales), and logged out through the computer. If there isn't a computer, a one-write receipt system should be in effect to serve a similar purpose.

Your consultant or accountant should be able to help you set up an appropriate internal control system, but the system will usually involve using a common sense, staff dependent, segregation of function. If the accountant can't or won't advise you (or wants to charge an extra fee), call a practice consultant who specializes in veterinary practice management, knows the veterinary profession's chart of accounts, and can help establish a practice-specific internal control system; the peace of mind alone is worth the investment. Quality veterinary practice consulting resources will usually offer the initial telephone consultation to a veterinary group administrator at no cost. There is no reason to remain at risk; act now, before it is too late for someone you trust.

Planning

Planning has multiple levels, ranging from technical manuals and personnel policies to the annual program-based budget that supports the one-year marketing plan and the one-year/three-year/five-year business plan that supports the owners desire for a community market niche. Planning can be top-down, but retreats that include all the managers is far better for creating ownership within the team; the group administrator acts **only** as the facilitator of these retreats. This is also a great technique for a single-facility practice.

In most situations, the veterinary practice's annual planning process should start three to six months (nine months for the group administrator) before the beginning of the budget year. Some practices meet quarterly and work four quarters in the future all the time. It seems to be more effective to strategically adjust for next winter immediately following this winter. For example, a target mailing to promote the value of the new isoflurane capability for all dogs over eight years of age with a "++" dental condition would require all medical records to have these factors recorded. Likewise, targeting all cats that have gained or lost 10 percent body weight (about one pound) in one year would require that every cat be weighed and the data recorded.

The planning team should include the owners, the doctors, all the key managers, and the bookkeeper. The use of a knowledgeable (but detached) facilitator is often critical to effective resolution of conflict situations; this is why we recommend the group administrator serve as the facilitator. The facilitator could also be a trusted consultant or even the practice CPA, if the accountant is knowledgeable about prospective planning (not just postmortem fiscal analysis). The group administrator, however, works with the individual manager all year, looking at programs and procedures, and is best suited for asking the right questions when the practice players get to brainstorming and dreaming.

Putting It Together

Multiple fiscal concerns have not been discussed here for many reasons, the least of which is the practices' lack of practice familiarity with the economies of scale potential in veterinary medicine in this decade. This is in the purview of the group administrator. The group administrator also is skilled in trend assessment and can balance the practice's trends against the expectations, the community demands, and the business skill of the healthcare delivery team. The fiscal management concerns of any facility within the group administrator's oversight should be addressed by a preoperational feasibility study, a baseline period, an expansion/sequencing impact priority list, as well as supporting information factors. The group administrator should address these management concerns with a knowledgeable financial planner, establish an investment plan, and integrate the return on investment (ROI) proceeds into operational and retirement planning.

The positioning required to make diversification possible can be initiated today by simply deciding to use the same hands-off management skills described above within your existing practice. Group-administrators-in-training will empower their staff, assist their confidence and knowledge levels whenever possible, and watch the results of their joint efforts. If this approach doesn't work in your existing practice, there are mixed messages being sent to the staff: they do not believe there will be a real change. This is a factor of practice culture, which may or may not be part of the group-administrator-in-training area of influence. The bottom line is that any perception is real to the person who holds it, and these perception factors must be overcome before progress and diversification can occur in any practice or group complex.

As is frequently said, you climb a mountain one step at a time. A skilled leader focuses the team's efforts on the next step, not on the top of the mountain. A great leader also understands that it is the grain of sand in the shoe, not the height of the step or mountain, which prevents success from occurring. Start the diversification process by eliminating the grains of sand that irritate the middle managers and paraprofessional staff, then start focusing on the steps up the mountain.

"Management du Jour" and Current Literature

Carpenters have the right tool for the right job, and sports figures have the best equipment available, but nothing *replaces the experience of life and hard work to get the job done right.*
—Dr. T.E. Catanzaro

We do consulting for a living. It is our full-time job. Everyone who contacts us wants an immediate cure for syndromes that have taken years to develop. They want that magic injection that every client thinks we have in the practice refrigerator, the one that will cure anything. We tell our clients not to believe everything they read, including what we write. Although I have written and contributed to numerous books on veterinary health care and on veterinary management issues, I still say, **"Don't believe everything you read!"**

All journals want the short article with the quick message. None are written for the group administrator. I know; I abbreviated my journal articles to the point that I had to write several books to tell the rest of the story. The journals and most readers want a cure that relieves the symptoms rather than one which attacks the causes of the disease. How many staff members have said, "and this too shall pass," after their manager or veterinarian has returned from a continuing education management conference? How many dedicated team members have become frustrated and disillusioned when they put their best efforts behind the theory du jour only to see it fail or have the management lose interest and start a new set of cures? This, my friends, is the environment that a group administrator walks into every time he/she decides to try expanding their business into new veterinary practices.

Management issues are complex, and good administrators know there is not one cookbook solution to fit all practices. Reputable administrators must first identify the strengths inside the practice, then build on them to capture community opportunities. There is rarely a single answer to a multifaceted practice challenge. Management fads are not bad, they are an evolutionary process that brings companies and practices to higher levels of awareness. For the group administrator (practice leadership) who integrates the fad into a well-established, annual practice plan, there is growth and development. Practices where managers and owners blindly pick a gimmick du jour often lose staff (e.g., Bottom-Line Sales Staff Beaters, Inc.), clients (e.g., Fee Boosters, Inc.), and their competitive advantage (e.g., Give It Away for Free and They Shall Come). And more importantly, they lose net practice income! The problem facing veterinary practices today is not the multitudes of management systems available, it is how to choose wisely from them. This ability to choose wisely is the bag of tricks that a good group administrator must bring to the negotiation table.

The Future Tense: The Stress of Change

Tense, as in stress, abounds when embarking on new ideas; a group facilitator is running a three-ring circus on any given day. Veterinarians generally want a guarantee of success before they start. In fact, fear of failure prevents practice growth more often than a lack of ability. As a matter of record, on most every consultation we have done during the past decade, the staff has always had some great ideas that have gone unheeded. Stress is often preceded by boredom, and that is not how a doctor ever started his/her first practice. Remember the energy levels, the commitment, and the hustle when the focus was on the front door swinging rather than on the bottom line of the income statement? Those were the days when each provider felt good stress, that pressure to achieve a new level of service, a new level of practice performance, for the benefit of others as well as him/herself. The savvy group administrator must restore that feeling in every provider, doctor, nurse, technician, receptionist, all the way down to the animal caretaker!

THE EIGHT-STEP SUCCESS PLAN

1. *Know who they are and what they stand for!*

   If it does not feel right, they are not ready for it. If they cannot be proud of doing it, then don't let it happen. Build on the strengths that have gotten them to the place where they lost their vision.

2. *Learn from their past.*

   Know where the strengths are in each staff member, and determine why certain ideas did not work. Was the practice climate not ready for change, or was it just the wrong idea at the wrong time?

3. *Know what others have done.*

   When other practices flounder, determine why. Empty parking lots may mean a high drop-off trade, so don't assume the worst until you know the facts.

4. *Make the new commitment with commitment!*

   Commit the resources and shout the new programs from the roof tops—if you don't have clear programs, you don't have a system which others can endorse.

5. *Communicate clearly where they are going.*

   Set measurable and achievable goals before starting on the road to change. Address doubts honestly and in a timely manner. Have clear milestones for success measurements, so the direction and pace can be celebrated en route.

6. *Create your own environment.*

   Do not overpromise then underdeliver. All new theories have old foundations, but any practice can move forward with fundamentals. Create words and programs that apply specifically to each practice, even if you must invent them.

7. *Have clear and achievable expectations.*

Know what is realistic, know what can be changed, and know who can attain the new level of performance. Have both short-term goals and long-term objectives, so success can come early and often.

8. *Just do it!*

Hoopla and hype are not needed, but dedication and loyalty to the team and clients are essential. Value is based on patient advocacy and client-centered service, not noise.

The critical factor for every management-du-jour idea is screening by the group administrator. Most practices take days to screen applicants for a single position within their practice, but they'll read about a new management gimmick and set everyone on their ears trying to make it fit the practice. An involved group administrator will start every management review (gimmick review) with a clear and concise statement of the practice core values and mission focus; more specifically, the group administrator will know what the practice needs to achieve **before** the review starts. In the *strategic assessment*, the group administrator must determine what the practice strengths are and what makes the team feel proud, and he/she will keep those features in mind as he/she fashions a strategic response. Good administrators will then do an assessment of other veterinary healthcare providers in their community (not pet food sales agents) and determine what the clients in the community want from their veterinary medical providers. In the *strategic response* process, the administrator matches the practice strengths to the community needs, then adds or expands the healthcare services in that area, as appropriate.

Ethics: Doing the Right Things

We awaken in others the same attitude
of mind we hold toward them.
—Dr. T.E. Catanzaro

USA Today ran a cover article about doing things wrong. I read it with great interest, and then realized that the problem was not leaders doing things wrong; it was leaders **not** doing the right things. Look at the list of unethical behaviors, which was developed by interview and survey of over 1,300 American workers:

TOP FIVE UNETHICAL BEHAVIOR ACTIONS
- Cut corners on quality assurance factors
- Covered up inappropriate incidents
- Abused or lied about sick days
- Lied to or deceived customers (clients)
- Put inappropriate pressure on others

We have seen the recent findings against insurance companies who misrepresented their products to senior citizens and must make amends. The companies blame this on their salespeople, but every insurance policy ever issued is reviewed by the underwriters—what was their charter? We have seen practice owners blame errors on a technician or receptionist, who was just following policy of the practice. We see practice managers (never call these people leaders) blaming the changes in their business flow on the other practices in town, or on the supersize pet stores in the area. Such managers don't accept as simple fact that if you are meeting the client needs, they will not go elsewhere! The group administrator must immediately reverse these trends whenever they are found, or they will be seen by the participating practices as ineffective administrators (remember the traditional veterinary management assessment approach is to always blame the other guy).

Ethics start at the top of any organization, and the group administrator must understand that the staff builds its perceptions of the practice ethics from the tone set by the owners and bosses (seldom will these people be considered *leaders* if the image they present is covert or unethical behavior). The practice owner who skims cash never trusts his staff. The doctor who lies to clients always believes the staff members are lying to him/her. The doctor who is unsure of a diagnosis and guesses at a treatment protocol, rather than offering and conducting the needed diagnostics, always suspects other practices in the area of just treating symptomatically. The doctor who does not trust nurse technicians to do what they were trained to do is often the same doctor who does not have the confidence to tell clients what is needed for the animal. This is also the doctor who X-rays the clients' wallets and makes decisions for the clients—covertly! Bioethics are involved in every euthanasia situation, every ear crop and tail dock, and most oncology prognoses (treatment discussions); when a doctor rationalizes less than quality healthcare delivery, the staff receives a confused message. Medical records must reflect needed care (❑) and client responses inside the "need box": waiver (*no way—ever*) = W, defer (*maybe next time, later*) = D, appointment (after pay day) = A, and "do it" = X. Actions are initialed by whoever did the treatment or process, and episodes are signed by the attending veterinarian; accountability is essential! A look at the top 10 factors in the *USA Today* survey that may trigger unethical behavior may make the picture clearer to the veterinary practice team.

TOP 10 FACTORS CAUSING UNETHICAL BEHAVIOR
- Need to meet sales, profit, or budget goals
- Little or no recognition of achievements
- Politics within the workplace
- Poor internal communications
- Balancing work and family
- Poor example by the top management
- Work hours—work load
- Lack of management support
- Personal financial worries
- Insufficient resources to get the job done right

In the *USA Today* survey, cited above, of 1,324 workers, 57 percent said they felt more pressure to be unethical than they had five years ago and 40 percent said pressure has increased over the past 12 months. Retail stores now plan to lose more to employee theft than to customer theft. Surveys show that entry-level restaurant and fast food workers admit to stealing an average of $239 per year in cash and merchandise. Some try to rationalize this by pointing out that our forefathers were the dregs of the earth and were sent or escaped to the United States to get out of prison or flee incarceration. I don't buy this! Good group administrators do not buy this. Veterinary providers must be beyond reproach in healthcare delivery, which means the leadership, including the group administrator, must set the tone not only in bioethics but also in community- and practice-related ethical behavior.

The expectation of unethical behavior is what disturbs me. In this same survey, 74 percent of the men and 78 percent of the women state that they feel their families have been neglected to some extent due to workplace pressures. Seventy-three percent believe that more open dialogue would help curb unethical behavior, and 71 percent say they need to see a more serious commitment by management. These numbers look low to me. These are the unmet needs of most every veterinary practice team member in America. It is the uncommon leader who dedicates adequate time to open feedback, meaningful ethics discussions, and commitment to the staff supporting the daily veterinary practice activities. For the group administrator, the pursuit of excellence must start with building the team; setting the example and creating a safe environment are critical support elements of this equation.

What does all of this mean to a veterinary practice administrator? In simplest terms, in trying to keep the lions from the door, some practices are

- Making exceptions to what they really believe in while trying to get the books to balance. The group administrator must bring the reality of the team back into focus with the providers.

- Replacing leadership with gamesmanship. The group administrator must bring the "game" back into focus with the providers.

- Grasping at straws and confusing their staff members. The group administrator must bring the "core values and mission focus" back into forefront with the providers.

- Controlling expenses into oblivion, and not paying enough to keep the good staff members because of either the financial greed or business unawareness of the ownership. The group administrator must bring the reality of the team back into focus with the providers.

The people who have joined veterinary medicine, from the doctor, to the nurse technician, to the receptionist and animal caretaker, have all joined the practice because of a calling of sorts. There must be an underlying value or trait that makes a staff member want to persevere. The group administrator must bring the reality of the team back into focus for the providers, then find the traits, beliefs, and values that motivate the staff and use them as a foundation for rebuilding the specific practice in question.

The dynamic group administrator of any practice must awaken the lions within, instead of fearing those at the door. He/she must lead by example, must redefine or realign the values that drew the team to this profession, and must nurture the team harmony. In short, leadership is a new way of life—think about it! Go now, and learn to be a knight among the camp followers.

L Listening—to others, attentively, and with an open mind

E Ethics—to do the right things, for the right reasons, at the right time

A Ambition—goals, imagination, and vision, backed by ability

D Desire—enthusiasm, drive, and determination to make things better

E Example—role models, ideals, honesty, common sense, and hard work

R Respect—for others, self, clients, patients, and life

S Self-esteem—poise and belief in self, nothing to "prove" to others

H Heart—empathize, nurture, and encourage

I Innovation—energy and ability to see things in a new way

P Patience—slow to criticize, quick to praise

CHECKLIST FOR MULTIPLE BOSS READINESS

Not everyone is made to be comfortable with becoming a group administrator, and not everyone has the knowledge and skills to become a contract manager to multiple practices. This checklist is a future tense review, not of your ability, but of your attitude; not of what is, but rather, of what you think can be. *The phraseology is based on the assumption that you have read and retained the subject matter provided in this text and in the texts listed at the beginning of this book.* Have fun with this, and start thinking about what you will do in the new millennium!

	I can do it!	Not for me.
I am willing to pursue education needs.	____	____
I am willing to pursue the CVPM credential.	____	____
I believe in the benefits of organized peer review.	____	____
I am willing to pursue the ACHE diplomate status.	____	____
I understand the operational principles of all three volumes in the ISU Press series, *Building the Successful Veterinary Practice.*	____	____
I can be HIGH I-S on the D-I-S-C Behavior Profile.	____	____
I am a HIGH D but can be HIGH I-S if I try.	____	____
I know the difference between leadership and management, and I am a leader of others.	____	____
I use the 14 leadership skills without thinking now.	____	____
I can build a program-based budget with doctors.	____	____
I can read an income statement and balance sheet.	____	____
I can determine variances by trend analysis.	____	____
I know that performance planning is far more effective than performance review/appraisal.	____	____
I use the leadership styles of directive training, persuasion, and coaching **before** ever attempting delegation.	____	____
I use effective teaching "discovery" daily.	____	____
I am using continuous quality improvement daily.	____	____

	I can do it!	Not for me.
I understand the need for barrier busting from the leadership skill *personal relationships*, and do it!	____	____
I like to give others credit for implementing my ideas.	____	____
I am willing to take blame for the staff mistakes.	____	____
I accept first mistakes as a form of personal training failure, not as a middle manager shortfall.	____	____
I believe in hearing the caring intentions **before** evaluating staff/doctor suggestion(s).	____	____
I am willing to get work done through others.	____	____
I want to develop others through work.	____	____
I believe in building my own replacement(s).	____	____
I know the doctor is not always right, but also understand the doctor is **never** wrong!	____	____
I sincerely believe any blaming abdicates the accountability for resolution; we do not play the blame game in conflict resolution.	____	____
I am willing to train the trainers in each facility and, maybe, put myself out of work.	____	____
I have conducted a council of clients.	____	____
I understand the effective use of outpatient nurses and nurse-client follow-up linkages.	____	____
I understand and use the "3Rs" in travel/circle sheet headings—to include computer linkages.	____	____
I know how to do internal promotions to produce peace of mind in veterinary medical clients.	____	____
I can disagree without making others wrong.	____	____
I know how to give truth with compassion.	____	____
I now realize that this checklist was developed just to check my attitude and mental flexibility, as needed for dealing with multiple practices!	____	____

4 Hiring a Group Administrator

*Strange how much you've got to know
before you know how little you know.*
—Anonymous

A Historical Perspective

As a consultant, the above quote of unknown origin speaks volumes. The history of veterinary practice management is as old as the profession. Noah had to do a space allocation survey just to float his boat with the original critters. I selected the veterinary management programs of the past decade for two reasons: (1) we have evolved and (2) Veterinary Forum asked me to keep it short and concise.

The Era of Paper

The 1980s were the era of paper. By 1984, one of the first great snowfalls of paper occurred when computer vendors showed people how to send multiple reminders (remember the 40 percent—50 percent—60 percent standard for first—second—third reminder effectiveness?). In 1985 and 1986, the clinic brochure became an important gimmick for promoting a practice, but many practices made them rule books rather than client solicitors. This problem still exists today at many practices.

Also in the mid-1980s, expense control became another paper-based art form. Expense control made national expense averages an easy item to publish, and since expenses were seldom aligned with income, net income was never discussed. Average client transaction (ACT) and gross revenues became the management gimmicks, and the pursuit of net income suffered. Expense control is something like taxation; only Congress believes we can be taxed into prosperity! We have started a new trend by providing a new look at program-based budgeting (Owen McCafferty, CPA, and I started the Catch the Wave seminars to share program-based budgeting in the mid-1990s, and like most new ideas, it was soon being copied profession wide). The expense control focus has continued for a full decade, and the veterinary medical profession is just now learning that there are alternatives (such as income centers and programs). In 1987, hospital newsletters had a flurry of activity but then fell into disuse because they didn't elicit immediate client reactions. Newsletters add to the six exposures **required** to get a yes action from someone who **already** knows they need something (over a dozen exposures in a short duration are required to get a yes response when people are not aware that they need something). To this day, many practices have not integrated their mailing program with internal promotion programs, and the program effectiveness is, in fact, below expectations in these cases.

By the time we got into 1988, when I wrote my very first medical record article for *AAHA Trends*, sample forms were becoming a viable practice management aid. AVMA was presenting their Marketing Strategies seminar with a full book of forms and checklists. During 1989, at AAHA, we developed break and stick labels to ensure pictures and formats could be quickly attached to a set of progress notes without ink pad or stamp. The stickers came in colors, and even included euthanasia releases and surgical summaries. These devices were soon available from AVLS, Petcom, PAL, and multiple other vendors. The sticker and form wars were upon us.

Concurrent with the above, the veterinary profession was marked as a viable market for mass marketing (another paper flurry) by those generic California management firms. These are the same firms that cook-booked the dentists, optometrists, and chiropractors in the 1970s and into the 1980s, and they had decided the veterinary profession was ripe for the picking. They were right, and practice consultants both from within the profession and from the outside emerged. The bottom line was simple: most veterinary practices were so weak in management that anybody with any new idea could make a difference.

The New Visual Media

The era of the VCR was in full swing by 1990. Ancom had swapped their closed-loop systems for VCR machines, Hills was giving the machines away with nutritional training programs, and staff training VCR tapes were being developed by AAHA, vendors, universities, and many other sources. The client education VCR tapes were beginning to proliferate from many sources, but when AVLS learned that five to six minutes was a client attention span, they captured a market niche.

Concurrent with this increase in audio-visual stimulation, 1990 saw the emergence of strategic planning, although even at the prestigious Veterinary Management Institute (VMI) at Purdue, it was the last module rather than the cornerstone required for tactical planning in the first three modules. During the 1990–1991 era, a new AVMA seminar program was introduced, with an interactive seminar format; this new program applied strategic planning to a mixed animal practice. Maybe mixed animal practices were slow starters, but this interactive seminar and mixed animal case study was a significant turning point for those veterinarians involved with other than small animal exclusive practices.

The Feeling Years

The feeling years addressed the activities of the head rather than the eyes, ears, or paper of the previous programs. In 1991, a series of stress management seminars appeared; they addressed the question of how to handle the stress and burnout associated with veterinary practice. Old-timers also called this boredom or frustration, but in emerging practices, 60- to 80-hour work weeks caused what newer practitioners called internal stress. New graduates wanted more out of life than just a clinic and caseload.

In 1992, stress management evolved to time management, but it did not quite take hold. Time management, in its simplest form, is the sequencing of events, and practices were losing control of the sequence. Competition was increasing, and alternative hours were seen as a method for combating the dual income household's inability to come to the practice during the normal daytime hours.

To combat both these trends and the emerging competition within larger communities seen in 1992–1994, traditional veterinary practice management took a leap forward and called itself *change management*—if you can't beat them, then adapt. This change management effort took many forms, from an increase of board certified specialists in the private sector, to specialized cat practices, to specialty vaccination clinics within the operational scope of traditional practices.

It is interesting to note that three elements are required for change management to occur. First there must be dissatisfaction or discomfort with what is, and it must be channeled into a desire to change (is this stress management?). The second step is identifying the appropriate model from the alternatives that could be pursued (visualization?). The third factor is participative process, where people have steps to follow to get from where they are to where they want to be (the paper era reappears). Again, cost control creeps into the equation when the costs of the dissatisfaction, the participative process, and the model are required to stay below the benefits achieved. And people wonder why change management cannot be done alone; there must be a guide who has traveled the unknown trails of change to ensure the practice owner will not return to the tree trunk and hold on until the termites come and eat it away. This guide through change management is most often a consultant; a veterinary-exclusive, nationally respected, practice consultant is better than any general consultant, but most veterinary practices are so far behind the power curve, most any consulting firm can help them.

Integration

The current emerging trends prove that what has gone before is still important, but like the basic sciences in veterinary school, it took clinical experience to bring it all together. The use of a well-designed clinical form is critical for people who need to develop new habits, but caring should eventually replace the robotic response. The use of brochures, handouts, visual aids, VCR tapes and other continuing education resources, for staff and clients alike, is important for effective veterinary practice operations. Furthermore, understanding the trends, the stresses, and the strategic needs of the practice's community is critical for adaptation actions by any practice. The secret of success is the integration of all of the above resources.

There has been a recent Association movement toward total quality management (TQM by Deming, Juran, and Crosby) and continuous quality improvement (CQI by JCAHO and Catanzaro & Associates, Inc., web site: <www.v-p-c.com>), but the average practice leadership is not ready to release that much control. What veterinary practices will see as we enter the new millennium is a movement toward leadership and team building, but the skills of leadership will need to be built on caring, knowledge, and the appropriate attitude. Some will present team building as another quick fix idea, but like continuous quality improvement (CQI) or total quality management (TQM), team building requires a total reassessment of what has gone before and a leadership commitment to change the old habits and empower the team. True leadership means assigning accountabilities for outcomes, rather than building manuals for the process.

The profession will see the integration and consolidation of resources to make integration and leadership occur. Since 1994, our firm has been promoting, sometimes with Gates Hafen Cochrane Architects or Owen McCafferty Accounting, leadership and team building as components of our seminars. In 1995, we even hosted a seven-day leadership training seminar. In 1996, we presented with Owen McCafferty, CPA, the Catch The Wave seminars, a series of seminars on program-based budgeting, in which income and clients rather than accountants and expense control drive the budget. These are forms of consultant networking and integration of disciplines; if we can do it across disciplines, practices can do it within the discipline of veterinary healthcare delivery. Integration of the strengths of the team members requires understanding their specific characteristics and needs. It requires balancing task orientation with a concern for keeping the group together. It requires a total integration of all that went before, from group development, to styles of leadership, to effective teaching. It is trusting others!

Integration of management means new leaders will emerge, people who are not looking for the quick fix or the gimmick of the month. It will mean that corporate America will hold out an olive branch of integration and economy of scale, and practices will have the choice to take it or fan the fires of tradition. The traditional management elements will continue to be refined and shared, but as with the skilled clinician, it will be the integrated programs and the committed leadership which will provide the management successes as we approach the end of this decade.

Social Trends: The Impact of Addictions

*Addiction—a state characterized by an overwhelming
desire or need (compulsion) to continue the use of
something and obtain it by any means.*
—*Dorland's Medical Dictionary*

During the past decade, alarming trends in healthcare delivery integration and social mores have emerged. Current experts have identified six major addictions of this era: food, work, sex, money, gambling, and drugs. Some have invaded our elected officials, some have impacted the leadership of our associations, and others are within our own community and are tearing at the fabric of trust. While these are not happy thoughts, they are concerns within veterinary practice consulting, so let's look at each addiction as it affects the veterinary medical profession.

Food

Food is good stuff, and nice to have; it is an essential for life. But we are seeing changes, even to the point of the Delta Society Annual Awards Banquet serving salmon rather than chicken or beef. Junk food has increased, but so also has the awareness of the importance of eating right. Some people are into healthier eating. In companion animal veterinary practices, the number of clients who use premium food has risen to about 30 percent, or a number almost equivalent to the A category clients.

The two-martini lunch has disappeared, and in veterinary medicine, most doctors do not take any lunch, which sets a bad example for the staff. Although everyone needs a mid-day lunch break (it is the law in most states), smart practices stagger lunch times so the practice can stay open during normal lunch hours. A pizza and soda party (or some other more healthful menu) is still one of the best ways to entice the staff to practice client narratives.

Work

The American work ethic has changed, and it is especially evident in the healthcare professions. The new professional expectations are often blamed on the feminization of the profession, but that is not the cause. The new generation of young adults wants a more balanced life. Work for the sake of work has been replaced by work for the sake of relaxation. To some, relaxation means better benefits, to others it means longer vacations or flexible work hours, and to a few, it means greater play time. This is not right or wrong; it is simply a fact.

This new attitude is the bane of veterinary practices, especially with the tenured professional staff. Practices have traditionally been built by the vision of a single veterinarian, and when it comes to expanding, a capability wall is confronted. We most often see this when practices plateau at an annual gross of $350,000 to $450,000 and call us for help (we can often double this per doctor income level with the effective use of the paraprofessional staff). The owner does not know how to share the workload, and the staff waits to be told what is needed.

As consultants, we have to introduce leadership and team building into the management formula and teach the owner how to release control. Although doctors do not like to release control, doctor-held control is not needed for most facility operational needs.

Sex

Many have mentioned the feminization of the profession, but the fact is that women have entered the work place at different levels than in the traditional "good old boy" network. The American work force has gained a new awareness of women as equals; the "girls at the office" do not exist anymore. Women are physicians, bankers, and even construction workers. About the only job women have not pursued is towel boy in a men's Turkish bath, but with the current laws on the books, pursuing it would be legal.

The ethics of proper working relationships between men and women has often not been set by example, only by law. We have seen national scandals when core values and personal ethics are not in alignment. In veterinary practices, the neglect of the male-female relationship is common, mainly because of the doctor-driven standards of healthcare delivery. Most practices have more female staff than male staff, but the traditional owner is a man. But ownership is changing, and many female doctors have shown capabilities greater than those of their male counterparts, when given a chance. The trend toward greater female participation in the profession does not, however, reduce the stress within the practice caused by a female doctor's entry into a previously male position. Sometimes this is most evident within the practice's paraprofessional staff, when the staff cannot work with the new female doctor because the doctor and the staff don't think alike. Operationally, anything is possible if expectations are clear and there is only a single standard within the practice and work ethic.

Money

Interestingly, money is almost always in the top six concerns of healthcare workers, but in every human healthcare survey, it has **never** made it to number one, and it is seldom even in the top three. During Christmas shopping in the late 1990s, VISA reported charge purchases in excess of a billion dollars per day. Americans like to buy things, but they don't like being sold anything. The cost of play, even movie tickets, is getting more expensive. In Colorado, lift tickets are over $50 per day, just to slide down a hill on a couple of boards and break your leg or frost your toes. In 1998, as a marketing response to community pressures, the ski hills started to allow four unrelated people (but they had to be Colorado residents) to buy a four-person family season pass for $800. The ski resort operators became aware of the discretionary spending patterns of the local community. The addiction to money is obvious, since we are often evaluated by the cars we drive, the suits we wear, the vacations we take, or the restaurants we frequent; smart marketers allow the image to be continued and popularized, while addressing discretionary spending limitations.

In America, people can earn what they deserve, or what they believe they deserve. Their salary level is a status symbol to some and a measure of self-worth to others. In veterinary practice, compensation rates are generally too low to be either, so additional monies must be used as recognition or as forms of thanks for special efforts. A practice with a solid, program-based budget understands that the mission focus and core values are the foundation of healthcare delivery programs and that solid programs can allow staff to make contributions to excess earnings or extra savings. When a staff member can contribute to excess savings or increased earnings, he/she provides a caring veterinary practice leader with another method of finding more money for recognitions.

Gambling

We first saw the Las Vegas connection being effected by Atlantic City, then by Native Americans who take advantage of their federal status, and now by the river boat communities. Pirates, profiteers, or entrepreneurs, it doesn't matter, there are people who want to play to win. Lotteries have even spread through state governments as a way to finance civic projects. People want to take a chance.

Opening a new veterinary practice in a shopping center three blocks from an established, free-standing, veterinary hospital is gambling. The new practice is gambling that it can steal enough clients not to starve. I say *steal* because everyone who wants a veterinarian can get to one, so a new practice often tries to attract clients who are already going to another practice; that is a form of stealing. Some clinicians gamble on most every case, rather than offer the client the diagnostics required for a better treatment plan. Some practices even gamble on surgeries because they don't tell the client that a laboratory profile is needed before general anesthesia—so we have anesthetic misadventures.

Some practices think they have clout enough to stop major corporations, but whether they are consolidating hospitals or selling pet food, it is a gamble that seldom pays off. It is critical to look internally and adjust (cope) rather than to look outside and gamble that someone will resolve the community trends.

Drugs

The drug problem is significant. We have professionals arguing the merits of marijuana, Presidents who "smoke grass without inhaling," and a former Surgeon General who excused drug use by her own children. The addiction epidemic is getting worse (caffeine, nicotine, and chocolate are legal addictions, but they are still drug addictions). Prescription drug abuse is overt and covert. Some veterinarians even pre-print their DEA numbers on prescription pads to help diverters. Some practices don't care about utilization and do not track drug use unless it is controlled (acepromazine recreational use and ketamine overdoses have become more common).

As the veterinary medical resource for the 22-state Regional Prescription Drug Abuse Task Force, I was enlightened to hear what Texas, Missouri, Oklahoma, and other states plan to do. One approach shared is to visit humane shelters and city pounds and to determine the euthanasia methods utilized. If a veterinarian is leaving euthanasia medication for staff use, a fine potential exists immediately. The state DEA plan is to visit the suspected veterinary practice, track substance use, and be prepared to impose fines for the misappropriations, poor documentation, and loss of control found in the review process.

Regardless of feelings of entrapment, the laws of the land are clear: controlled substances must be controlled. Furthermore, ethically labeled drugs require ethical use; they must not be dispensed to anybody who wants an over-the-counter purchase. The diversion of specific drugs to some gym for bulking up with steroids is now a special attack point (Anabolic Steroid Act of 1990) in many communities, and some traditional, non-controlled, pain medications became controlled in 1997. To divert or abuse the professional responsibilities of a veterinary practice is a gamble, often one with a heavy fine. The penalty may be monetary (FDA or DEA), or it may affect the youth in the community. Environmental Protection Agency (EPA) violations, for example, pollute our community, and the generations who follow will pay the price. If we don't start to control ourselves, others will do it for us.

Plan of Action

As a hospital administrator or as a practice owner looking to hire a hospital administrator, you must be aware of the above addictions. They cannot be tolerated in a veterinary healthcare delivery system, and if they do exist, they are usually medical conditions which the practice's insurance must cover during resolution. Think positive—there are alternatives. For addictions and for other bad habits that already exist, in yourself or in others, there are five steps to clarify the problem as well as five steps to resolve it, but **achieve clarity first.**

Steps to Clarity

1. *Think of a problem, habit, or addiction.* Define the bad experience, everyday difficulty, or problem, habit/addiction.

2. *See yourself as a snapshot.* Pick out one moment you are not proud of and look at it as if was a snapshot of a younger you.

3. *Add a picture frame.* The snapshot is surrounded by a frame, an environment, and you must resolve the selection of that frame. What shape do you want the environment to be in for the snapshot frame?

4. *Make the snapshot and frame a work of art.* Reframe the snapshot with a better frame (environment) and reform the snapshot in a more artistic pose. Look at the potential and alternatives of the situation.

5. *Check the results.* Clear your mind, compare the original incident to the new picture and frame. Your feelings and standards may have changed during the reframing and reposing. If not, reframe the environment potentials and repose the snapshot of what you could be. Picture a better world until you find one that agrees with your feelings.

Steps to Resolution

One key item in a great leader's bag of tricks is this secret tool: **make people part of your resolution goal.**

1. *Choose a goal.* You have the right to choose the revised snapshot and the improved frame. Be specific in your thought pictures.

2. *Identify the resolution goal.* Have clarity in the resolution picture in your mind (see the five steps above), identify the feelings associated

with the better snapshot and better frame (environment); know where you are going!

3. *Decide on the people involved.* Think of the people who enter the environment which exists and which you have pictured, and identify which ones are necessary for the new resolution goal. Add sights, sounds, and smells whenever possible, even if you must expand the snapshot frame (environment). With whom do you need and want relationships en route to the resolution?

4. *Define how the key people relate to you.* If they are not in the fore-ground of the new snapshot, put them there. Relationships cause commitments when times are tough, and addiction resolution is the roughest when you redesign your environment. We all need help at this phase.

5. *Future planning.* Think of the time in the future when the revised snapshot and frame will be a reality, and accept that energy and sac-rifice will be required to make it a reality. Share the picture you have built with the key people in the picture, and make a pact that they will stay in the center of that snapshot until it is reality.

Postscript

As a consultant, I have seen addictions of many types, and they are most often associated with some form of co-dependency with those close to the addicted person. Addiction often destroys relationships with well-qualified management candidates, as well as with new asso-ciates. We cannot discuss hiring unless we look at the things that cause disasters in newly forming relationships. And that is most often an ad-dictive or compulsive behavior on the part of the employer and less of-ten, but also with some frequency, on the part of a middle manager or an administrator. Empathy does not mean sympathy, nor does it mean losing one's personal identity. The best friend to an addict is actually someone who won't make excuses and will not support the addiction; co-dependency is **not** allowed! The person who changes standards, ig-nores core values, or modifies his/her beliefs to meet an addict's need for blaming someone else won't be thanked until after the addiction is resolved, but those who weather the storm will be able to celebrate the sunlight. It is a nice feeling.

Establishing Personal Practice Priorities

Time management is simply the sequencing of events,
since we cannot control time; priorities are what make
the sequencing productive and meaningful.
—Dr. T.E. Catanzaro

Practice philosophy is simply a mission focus concerning what the ownership believes is the practice's basic reason for existence **and** what is delivered by the staff. In progressive practices, the practice philosophy, mission statement, vision statement, or whatever term is used to describe this statement, is generally restricted to less than 25 words. The *mission focus* on the other hand is not a statement; it is an application of the core values that were used to define the practice philosophy, vision, or mission statement. For instance, the three most critical practice goals for this year as well as the three most important long-range goals of the practice should be known by everybody. Once these bits of information are established, personal goals can follow.

Without a clear practice philosophy, core values, and known goals, it is very hard for any staff member to set realistic priorities without disrupting the veterinarian or manager. This "check-with-the-boss" system is common but very inefficient and frustrating. The area of individual responsibility varies with the practice, as does flexibility within the area of responsibility; the hospital administrator needs to have a comfort zone established with the practice ownership that allows for unilateral changes of these boundary systems. In the advanced practice management situation, the *what* (an output, outcome, or expected result) is all that is tasked by the boss, and the *how* is the responsibility of the staff member assigned the accountability for the results expected; the administrator is the coordinator of the agreements and time lines.

The perfect job description is a myth of veterinary practice. Staff members were not hired to do a job; they were each hired to solve problems in a specific area of practice. The simple fact is that daily veterinary practice is a series of problems. Even if it is not said, accolades and acknowledgment usually are restricted for those times when someone extends beyond the job description for the good of the practice. Pride in performance **only** comes when someone can exceed expectations; good administrators ensure expectations are set so there is at least a 60 percent success rate by the team members. This is the philosophy that has caused continuous quality improvement (CQI) to become so successful in human healthcare delivery environments.

Tasked Priorities

Following preordained priorities usually causes more problems than are solved; staff members need to be empowered to set priorities based on the environment of the moment and on the known protocols of practice (technical manuals). Personal priorities include harmony and, more important, happiness. If a staff member can't look forward to going into the practice, the first priority must be to change that attitude or to change his/her job (within or outside the scope of the practice). When addressing the attitude aspect of priority setting, evolving administrators must remember the following hints:

- Mix with critical people, and you learn to criticize. Mix with happy people, and you learn how to have enjoyment in your life.

- Mix with messy people, and your life becomes messy. Mix with organized people, and you learn how to become better organized.

- Mix with enthusiastic people, and you learn excitement. Mix with complaining people, and you learn how to look at life as a frustration.

- Mix with adventurous people, and you learn how to take risks. Mix with the timid, and you learn how to avoid change.

- Mix with status quo managers, and you learn how to stabilize a practice to death. Mix with leaders, visionaries, and change agents, and you learn how to meet changing community demands.

What these hints tell us is that we need to decide what we want from life and then choose our work style accordingly. You might believe that it will offend some other staffers within the practice, and that may be uncomfortable. But it is your life.

It is known that *change* requires three elements to be present in almost equal proportion: *dissatisfaction/discomfort* (with the habit, not with the person), *process* (acceptable methods) and a *model* (clear goals or outcome expectations). If you set priorities that address only one of the three elements, success will not be complete; more often, it will not be achieved. The other consideration in change management is choosing when to start the change process; the simplest answer is, "Live now! All you have is *now*."

The measures of our peace of mind and of our personal effectiveness are determined by how much we are able to live in the present moment. We cannot become distracted with what happened yesterday or what may happen tomorrow; we must be focused on what can be done today, at the present moment. CQI is based on increasing the pride in performance today so tomorrow may be made better by the effort.

Triage Requirements

Triage is defined medically as the sorting out and classification of casualties of war or other disasters, to determine priority of need and proper place of treatment. In the hiring process, ensure that every candidate understands that a healthcare administrator must be ready to deal with triage situations. Triage could be defined as standards of healthcare urgency applied to priority of care decisions, under limited resource conditions. Since I did triage as a medical administrator in Vietnam during 1967 and 1968, I will tell you it is applying core values to difficult life and death decisions that are impossible to resolve emotionally. Some reception areas are automatically classified as disaster areas, and some inpatient facilities become war zones when treatment modalities are questioned. But let's define emergencies as our first triage need; they can be client defined or practice defined:

- Everyone agrees that an animal hit by car or having a seizure is an emergency.

- Veterinarians agree that one dilated pupil on a valuable breeding animal indicates a need for early diagnostic work-ups on a priority basis.

- Clients who procrastinate on a health certificate until the day before a trip perceive an emergency situation.

- Whenever a client perceives an emergency, a healthcare provider must respect that perspective; the good news is that healthcare delivery can be assessed at higher rates for perceived emergencies.

A good receptionist deals with each of the above examples in the same caring, expeditious manner, since she/he realizes perception is reality. In reality, the ability to remain neutral during the search and sort effort often finds alternative resources:

- Triage health care by admitting walk-in patients with questionable health histories and letting the professional healthcare delivery team sort out the problems and re-contact the owner.

- Triage telephone emergencies by using such statements as, "Our doctor reserves from __ to __ to return client calls. What number will you be at during that time?" or "That is the type of condition that we feel should be seen immediately for evaluation so we don't miss subtle signs, can you come in at ___?"

- Triage front desk emergencies (other than admitting the patient) by routing the client/patient into an open examination room **or** rescheduling for a later time that day. Whatever option is chosen, the front desk staff must **always** stay cool and respond to what the client feels is needed for the pet.

- In high-density scheduling scenarios, the inpatient team takes all emergencies and walk-ins, which reduces stress on other staff members. This also allows inpatient fees to be assessed as needed.

The toughest triage decisions deal with pain, suffering, and death. We can treat pain, but we cannot treat suffering, whether in animals or owners. There should be a pain scoring system in place before a hospital administrator is even considered, and it must be a staff-wide standard of care. We must have empathy and compassion, but we cannot promise miracles. Since we must actively participate in killing animals (euthanasia), we must keep a strong grip on the humane and ethical basis (quality of life) for our decision making. Any veterinary healthcare administrator must accept this charter of active euthanasia as a term of employment. We often let this professional value system get clouded by breeders or unwanted offspring. Conscious decisions within the practice and subconscious values within the practice team do not always agree; open interstaff communications are critical to this triage concern.

Building for a Better Tomorrow

A tree as big around as you can reach starts with a small seed; a thousand-mile journey starts with one small step.
—Lao-Tse

Life is a building process. Today's efforts create tomorrow's results. No one has all the facts needed to make an error-free decision, so administrators must make decisions based on partial information using the core values and mission focus of the practice. Know what the core values and mission focus are before you start the hiring process. It does not matter whether you attack a nasty habit, spend an hour with the family, complain about the world, set goals, spend or save, take risks or avoid them, your decision is what makes the difference. Tomorrow starts with today, and yesterday can never be changed.

Before anyone has a party, he/she makes a list of needed supplies as well as a guest list. Before a person goes shopping, he/she makes a list, to make sure nothing is forgotten; it keeps the shopper on track and within known resources. The surprising thing is that fewer than 5 percent of the people ever use written lists to get their lives organized. Doesn't your celebration of life deserve as much written structure as we give to grocery shopping or partying?

CQI is based on making tomorrow better than today, but that first requires taking responsibility for today. If you haven't been given accountability, ask for it. Continuous quality improvement requires that each team member commit to personal excellence in whatever they touch or whatever touches their area of accountability. You can't change others, but you can often control your job satisfaction, especially when you accept that *you were not hired to do a job, you were hired to solve problems.*

You can influence the **pride** you have in your daily functions, and that pride is seen by clients as **quality**. When this process is translated into the CQI terms, we say that as you try to have more pride and harmony in your work, the practice will have more quality in the healthcare delivery perceptions of clients. Quality translates to the bottom line only because of the top line, clients: clients keep coming back to the practice. The staff is critical in this formula, so remember the team-building adage, *if it is to be, it is up to me.*

Compensation for Practice Managers

Leadership is action, not position.
—Dr. T.E. Catanzaro

The position of practice manager, hospital manager, business manager, office manager, hospital administrator, or contract practice manager (with or without an administrative assistant) means different things to different folk. Remember the definitions we listed at the beginning of this text:

- *Hospital administrator*. The hospital administrator has complete authority over the business and operations of the practice in concert with the owners/board, has final authority in fiscal decisions, and is the supervising agent of all facility services, products, personnel, and quality assurance. The hospital administrator is also the coordinating agent for medical protocols short of therapeutic decisions, continuity of care, and all functions of a practice manager and an office manager.

- *Practice manager*. The practice manager manages the business activities and practice internal promotions, possesses all the knowledge of an office manager, and has direct authority and decision-making responsibilities over all business aspects of the practice.

- *Hospital manager*. This position is not defined by VHMA, but is generally similar to practice manager.

- *Business manager*. This position is not defined by VHMA, but is similar to office manager with heavier bookkeeping and budget monitoring roles and fewer staff supervision functions.

- *Office manager*—Office manager is the entry position into middle management in most hospitals. He/she is involved in daily accounting, accounts receivable, banking, schedule coordination, purchasing, accounts payable, training, directing the front office staff, and client relations.

- *Group administrator (contract practice manager)*. The group administrator is a management person outside the staff structure who is on contract to the practice. He/she manages multiple practices within a geographic region and has the proven knowledge and skills of a practice manager or higher.

- *Administrative assistant*. This title is generally reserved for a staff person working within a single practice but trained and directed by an outside contract management person. The administrative assistant is jointly supervised by the contract practice manager and the facility owner.

Methods for Computing Compensation

The title is not as important as trust; responsibility is not as important as the accountability; and compensation is **always** negotiable;

these factors are all defined by the ownership. The job description in progressive practices, for managers/administrators, could simply read, "Solve/prevent problems and make continual quality improvements." The three basic methods for computing the manager's value to the practice (or compensation for performance) are

- *The Income Method.* Based on percent of gross (2–3.5 percent). For a savvy administrator, this is often set lower than normally desired during negotiations, and some form of quarterly recognition fee based on a portion of the excess net (e.g., 20 percent of the increase, or 20 percent over the balance sheet requirements) is added to the existing compensation.

- *The Market Method.* Based on worth of experience and knowledge: CVPM (VHMA), VMI (Veterinary Management Institute) theory course (AAHA), college degree(s) (education investment), Diplomate (board certified) of the American College of Healthcare Executives.

- *The Cost Method.* Divide the compensation required to live within the chosen profession by the charge hours available to get an hourly fee requirement. [The compensation figure is adjusted for costs, amortized equipment (five years), overhead, and taxes. For the charge hours figure, charge hours available in the year (usually 2,500–2,600) are adjusted for budgeted sick time, vacation time, continuing education, speaking engagements, etc., to get available hours in the annual schedule (usually 1,800–2,000).]

For example, under the *income method*, a two-doctor, $450,000 gross, companion animal practice can afford about 3.5 percent for the manager, or $15,750 (poverty wage). However, with a quarterly excess net of about $8,000, the manager gets an additional $1,600 per quarter or about $6,400 per year added to the base, for an annual compensation of $22,150. This is a reasonable number, since a two-doctor practice can produce $600,000 or more in a well-managed operation (which would increase the base to more than $21,000). Under the *market method*, you negotiate the worth of experience and knowledge, and if necessary, get the VHMA annual salary survey data for your region (but you may not like being average). For the *cost method*, let's start with the following example: $50,000 compensation + $5,000 costs + $35,000 facility overhead expenses + $10,000 taxes (payroll, etc.) = $100,000; then divide the $100,000 cost of living in the profession by

2,000 available hours to get the $50/hour break-even rate to be assessed for services.

The bottom line for a veterinary practice consultant is that no one in a leadership role should hold out for a hefty base salary. Each level **deserves** a minimum living value, with a board certified hospital administrator starting at $62,000, a practice manager with a CVPM starting at about $45,000, and an on-the-job trained (OJT) office manager starting in the mid-20s. These numbers do vary with the section of the country (e.g., the Northeast and southern California will most always be more expensive, while salaries in the Southeast and Midwest may be lower).

What Managers Are Really Paid

As competition increases in the veterinary market, everyone from the solo practitioner to public corporation vice presidents is searching for ways to survive and succeed in these changing times. Their prosperity often depends on qualified managers and administrators who have the knowledge, skills, and the attitudes to make others successful; vision, core values, and sound business judgement are foundation elements. From the office manager to the hospital administrator, veterinary managers influence your practice's success. What salary and benefits do these supervisors receive?

All veterinary managers and administrators work similar hours (42 to 55 hours a week). When it comes to pay, there is a greater variance. Entry-level managers earn an average annual salary of $26,000 (area dependent), while experienced practice managers make closer to an average of $33,000. Veterinary hospital administrators earn an average salary of $45,000 to $55,000. The group administrator who charges **only** $1,000 a month for a half day every week with the practice's team but centralizes fiscal administration, inventory management, human resource procurement, and staff development for six practices will earn $72,000 a year.

Supplemental compensation methods vary greatly between practices, with many managers getting a cut of gross or a share of savings. Savvy administrators will hold out for a share of the change in the net, since it encompasses both savings and program enhancements. Practice owners must liberally address benefits such as disability insurance, medical/dental family plans, retirement funds, and other profit-sharing opportunities when looking for skilled administrators. Nearly all managers and administrators deserve an aggressive continuing education allowance, since continuing education is critical in a CQI environment. Look at this sliding scale of opportunities:

- *Office managers* should be fully funded in the local veterinary management group or be provided with annual registration and per diem to a state-level veterinary medical management meeting. Payment of dues to VHMA is highly encouraged.

- *Practice managers* should be fully funded in the VHMA, registered on VIN management access, and provided with annual registration and per diem to a regional-level veterinary medical management meeting.

- *Hospital administrators* should be fully funded in the VHMA and CVPM certification process, and the practice(s) should provide fiscal support for the administrator to hold office in the VHMA or local veterinary management group. The veterinary hospital administrator needs to be provided with annual registration and per diem to a national veterinary medical management meeting.

Non-monetary Factors

Besides compensation factors, veterinary managers and administrators need to feel confident about their respect, responsibility, and recognition levels; these all support a feeling of trust and job security. Veterinary practice managers and hospital administrators deserve an opportunity to invest money in practice ownership, even if it is just a portion of the practice, such as the grooming, boarding, or boutique operations. "[E]very manager should have reward opportunities that aren't title-related" (Peter F. Drucker, *Management: Tasks, Responsibilities, Practices*, New York: Harper Business, 1993).

A real healthcare administrator and practice leader must be prepared to both receive the rewards of practice success and suffer the anguish of practice failure. I use the term *leader* because that is what these turbulent times require. Leaders use situational leadership, since they realize their job is to accomplish the mission (task) through other people. Managers, by contrast, have programs and projects and emphasize the *proper process* for themselves and others. They control expenses, establish policies and procedures, and assign jobs (tasks) as needed. They take credit and give blame, while a leader gives credit and accepts blame. A leader realizes that the team is strength and that the outcome is what really counts. A leader has confidence in his/her team and shares rewards, gives recognition, and nurtures each individual as a special practice asset. A leader accepts accountability for the results of his leadership.

Managers who desire a hefty base pay are not likely leaders; they want a compensation that is guaranteed, regardless of performance. This is a warning flag. Practices need to pay for performance, not promises. True leaders trust in their people and the capabilities of the team to make improvements, solve problems, and increase client services (and thus increase the liquidity). A good healthcare administrator will ask for a percentage of success and then ask the team to excel. Such administrative leaders will establish expectations and offer individualized training to make it possible for the practice to reach those expectations.

Aids for the New Administrator

Veterinary practices are getting larger and more complicated each year. More are reaching the economic point where they can afford a hospital administrator (3–3.5 percent of the gross). Many practices are promoting from within, and that is where problems often begin. The great technician or receptionist is not necessarily a qualified hospital manager; we must take time to help these people make the transition into their new practice roles.

Some common reasons given by new managers for failure or inability to assume the job role include the following:

- They lacked the common-sense experience needed to succeed in spite of the practice system.

- They did not know what was expected of them or where their limits and responsibilities were.

- They were given the responsibility for the tasks without being given the related authority.

Common Sense

This short description is designed to convince the practice owner that the new practice manager, hospital administrator, or group hospital administrator has the skills, capabilities, and experience to be an outstanding leader. The skills and capabilities the candidates have used to get where they are today can be used to improve the practice's position tomorrow. But remember, if you are satisfied with what you did to get where you are today, you will stagnate; stagnation is stasis, and in life stasis means death. Practices should hire a manager or administrator because they want to move to the next level, and want to allow the doctors to return to patient care. Veterinarians doing management chores should be paid $10 per hour, whether they are owners or employed associates; doctors are healthcare team leaders, not pencil pushers. Some of the skills and capabilities doctors learn while building a practice allow them to be trainers of others, but sometimes even those capabilities need to be refined or redirected to make the administrator's role work for the practice. Owners looking to hire management expertise into a practice, or even develop it from within, must

- *Allow the management team to be hands-on managers.* Know your people and keep communications open. Give them the trust they deserve, but do not abdicate your responsibilities to healthcare delivery in the practice. Stay informed about their projects and their client contacts; know what they'd like to be doing within the practice. Mentor the senior manager or administrator and stay out of the daily operational maintenance functions. Go deliver care to patients, talk to clients, or review the current literature on the Internet (if you cannot surf the net, learn how soon, it is a requirement for professional survival in the new millennium).

- *Allow managers to win.* This does not mean playing to avoid losing. Willingness to accept sensible risk is vital to any manager's success. Qualified healthcare administrators will tell you that only 40 percent of the great ideas survive, 20 to 40 percent will die within 90 days, and the balance will fail unless adjustments or major changes are made during the implementation process.

- *Trust and follow your instincts.* Do your homework before offering advice or making decisions, but also have the courage to accept the manager's convictions. If the manager believes he/she is right, go with it. When a manager brings you a problem, and as the "big boss" you ask for two alternatives, if either would work, let the manager make the choice, and be sure you praise the effort.

- *Build and cherish relationships.* Ensure your management team is allowed and encouraged to network with managers and administrators from other practices and with business leaders in the community. Learn from others who have tried it before. Allow them to build practice accomplishments over the long term.

- *Put issues into proper perspective.* Remember the practice core values and mission focus that drove the goals and objectives for the year, as well as your personal goals. Ensure that the administrator or manager can depend on **your** consistency and support. These are the guidelines that often make the tough decisions easier.

- *Don't expect help from anyone else.* Everyone has his/her own agenda, and some individual agendas may not coincide with those of the practice or your leadership team. Don't confide vulnerabilities to practice associates; it is okay to ask for help toward a practice objective, but do not expect unilateral effort from others unless you are leading the team.

- *Cultivate self-esteem.* The theory of self-fulfilling prophecy really holds true for new managers and administrators. Whether they think they can or they think they can't, it will come true; if they believe in their own success, it will happen. As a practice owner, your positive mental attitude will make jumping the hurdles in practice operation easier—use future think!

Delegating Decisions

As a practice leader, realize that decisions must be made when they are needed. New practice managers or administrators who are insecure, however, often opt to wait until the owner/veterinarian is available, even though the responsibility to act has been assigned to them with the manager title. This management situation leaves hired team leaders with two grim options:

- Stick out their necks and endanger their positions by making the decision themselves and suffering the wrath of the boss.

- Miss a potentially great opportunity and end up looking ineffective.

I wish it was as easy as waving a magic wand and telling each new manager that the veterinarian releases control by the simple act of hiring someone to manage the practice; that is not true in most cases. Most practices are built with the sweat and tenacity of a single veterinarian or, as practices get larger, two or three veterinarians. These small practices are built by process control. The challenge is that most veterinary hospitals hit a wall at $500,000, plus or minus $200,000, unless there is a leadership awakening.

The reverse side of the doctor who cannot give up control is the older doctor who hires an administrator and abdicates (even disappears in some cases). There are steps a savvy manager can take to tame the absentee boss and do his/her job more effectively:

- *Keep a clear list of what ifs.* When you can pin the veterinarian down, discuss the common hypothetical situations that you think could arise. Sound out how they should be handled and by whom.

- *Maintain a running list of questions and issues.* As the staff and you think of situations, write them down in a sequential list. At the next meeting, you won't waste time sorting through your notes or trying to remember what happened that needs discussion.

- *Set up a regular meeting.* Make it clear to the practice owner or the managing veterinarian that you need a chance to talk over current projects on a weekly basis.

- *Establish emergency procedures.* Find out who can make the professional decisions when the owner is unreachable. Determine what decision latitude you have in pet emergencies, in client emergencies, and in staff emergencies. Establish which decisions the boss wants done by consensus in his/her absence, and what decisions **must** be held for the owner.

- *Ask for prototypes.* Models of budgets, schedules, presentations, and manuals can answer many questions even before you think of them, especially the first time you tackle a new project for the practice.

- *Talk to others in the practice.* Find out how others in the practice have effectively dealt with the owner/veterinarian. Use techniques that have been successful before; you will probably get the staff's moral support as an added benefit.

- *Make sure everybody knows that decision-making information is routed through you.* When given adequate time, especially in the early days of your management career, gather the decision data available, outline the options, and choose the one that seems best for you. Then present the data as information (process and organize the data personally) with the option you favored. You will save the practice owner or veterinarian time and energy as well as impress him/her with your ability to think critically and make decisions, while testing the waters for an okay.

- *Communicate creatively.* Find in-between time for meetings, on the drive to the next community meeting, over breakfast, while the owner waits for an airplane. Use fax machines to send questions to and get replies from the owner, practice consultants, or other experts who can assist you to succeed. The best method is to compose memos with options that can be simply checked off; phrase the options so that a *yes* or *no* can be a cause for action.

Service Skills

Service has become an obsession in the United States, mainly because it is an acceptable way to differentiate between professional practices, but also because it works. Few successful new managers can escape the demand to demonstrate increased sensitivity to clients, and such sensitivity must be seen as part of the manager's responsibility whether assigned or assumed.

An interesting fact is that within a veterinary practice, a new manager/administrator has at least three sets of clients. The first set owns pets and comes through the front door looking for help. The second set is the community that interacts with the practice, whether it is the elementary school seeking a speaker, the Society for the Prevention of Cruelty to Animals (SPCA), the animal control office, vendors, or just high school kids looking for a yearbook ad. The third set is the staff of the practice; they look to the manager for leadership and tough decisions that will help them provide quality service to the practice clients while giving them a good quality of life.

Some guidelines are provided below that apply to the application of the skills and capabilities discussed above. These guidelines can apply to receptionists, exam room communications, or personal interactions. Make them a lifestyle goal to help yourself become an effective veterinary practice manager:

- *Act genuinely interested in the concern of the client.* Never dismiss a question with an indifferent response; this includes stopping what you are doing, making eye contact, and paying physical attention to the person who asks the question. Being the focus for a solution for staff or clients is always a good manager's responsibility.

- *Don't abdicate the responsibility to make things right.* There is nothing more frustrating than to be shunted to another person when looking for help. If you can't help, take the problem from the client or staff member and promise to get back to them in a timely manner. Keep your promises; a manager's word is the cornerstone of leadership strength.

- *Listening is most important.* When someone tries to explain a frustration, listen for the gist of the problem. Often it underlies the words spoken, but it must be determined to resolve the frustration.

- *Keep cool and speak softly.* When all about you is going crazy, become the port in the storm that others can look to for guidance and sanctuary. By keeping your cool, speaking softly, and not making the knee-jerk decisions, you can be a stability factor in the practice.

- *Don't become impatient.* Many clients appear confused or just seem dumb. This is not unusual since they do not understand the science of veterinary medicine, the business of the practice, or the interactions of the staff. Many of the staff do not fully understand these factors either. Speak slowly and ask questions to clarify the problem before searching for alternatives.

Responsiveness is what differentiates the average manager (or practice) from the one that is perceived as better. The responsive service skills decrease complaints and dissatisfaction. Even in New York, where no one ever seems happy, complaints were reduced five-fold after a utility company gave its service operators training in customer service.

A new practice manager must prepare to be successful. Luck is often defined in management as the act of preparing to capture the opportunity as it quickly passes. If you decide to rely on luck in your new position, start preparing now and refine it daily. If you do not rely on luck, start preparing today and get better daily with additional hard work and research in management skills.

How to Train a Hospital Manager

The first two responses that come to mind are "with a whip and a chair" and the less extreme "by example." There are many management theories and a lot of nifty strategies, but the bottom line is that we need results. To get you started on the right track, here are some planning-to-plan ideas that have worked in the past:

- *Step One:* Define the job tasks of the hospital manager by outcome expectations and include not only time line expectations but also quantitative and subjective expectations.

- *Step Two:* Determine which responsibilities will be relinquished to the manager and develop a plan for transferring the authority and the resources required to accomplish the task within the given expectations.

- *Step Three:* Develop a list of expected milestones with intermediate objectives that are necessary to successfully complete the training plan for the new manager, so there will be interim recognition opportunities as the training progresses.

- *Step Four:* Make a list of management and leadership skills that the person must possess to accomplish the first three items utilizing only on-site training by existing staff. Determine what supplemental knowledge or skills may be required.

- *Step Five:* If step four does not give you the knowledge or confidence needed to be successful, be ready to seek assistance from outside trainers, continuing education experiences, or a consulting team with the required skills needed to make the action occur as planned.

The above planning-to-plan steps are critical. The responsibilities of the new hospital manager must be supported by the authority to make unilateral decisions for the good of the practice. These decisions must not be undermined by the practice owner, his/her spouse, or the tenured team members. This delegation of authority allows the veterinarian to return to the examination room and the clients and leave daily operational concerns to the hospital manager.

While there are many management theories, the key to success is knowing what motivates the new hospital manager. If we know where his/her hot buttons are, we can punch them up to accelerate the learning curve. In the United States, the focus of motivation for healthcare employees is recognition. The focus of motivation differs from nation to nation, so beware of tips learned in Japan, England, or other forward countries. Recognition as a motivational factor is correlated strongly and positively with the perceived importance of the job, advancement opportunities, personal growth, and the expectations that successful task accomplishment will be rewarded and that personal effort will lead to successful task accomplishment. Our training plan must be based on the appropriate motivational factors to be successful.

Each practice is unique and each practice owner has personal preferences for relinquishing authority, but training must accent the need for group genius. Mere brainstorming with the staff for ideas will never evoke genius. The most effective managers and leaders understand that tasks are accomplished through the involvement of other people. The staff must become a team, and the team needs to focus on taking moderate risks to become comfortable with innovation. Positive valuing techniques need to be used. Instead of asking, "How do we fix the parking problem?", the team focus becomes, "How can we best improve the parking system?" The thoughts need to become "What if ... ?" or "Maybe we could ..." and extend beyond the customary limitations, ultimately moving to a vision of how things need to be in five years. The objectives and goals used to reach the vision must be based on a team consensus, and the hospital manager is critical to that process. If you are not yet willing to use a hospital manager in that role, you really don't want a true hospital manager; you want an extension of yourself—a gofer (a go-fer-this and go-fer-that employee who is under your control).

Team achievement skills are critical. You cannot deliver quality health care unless the whole team is involved. Team achievement results can be evaluated in terms of productivity improvement, but that is only one aspect of achievement. There will be many changes best measured in qualitative terms such as quality of work life and morale that also have a significant bottom-line impact. People will enjoy their work more, absenteeism and tardiness will decrease, and the leader becomes an approachable colleague rather than a threat.

The areas that need attention in most practices are those in the hospital administrator's sphere of influence.

- *Time management.* Very few practices really know how much time is spent doing which functions. A new hospital manager can become an expert in this area in a very short time.

- *Cost centers.* Determining the total cost of individual functions (to include equipment replacement) has generally not been done for each outpatient, inpatient, surgical, dental, and ancillary service.

- *Income centers.* By integration of time management results and cost center evaluations, income (+/− profit) centers can be identified for marketing efforts. This integration of information is a natural task for the concerned hospital manager who understands that personal efforts must cause savings or income to offset the new salary of the hospital manager.

- *Performance evaluations.* Transferring the 90-day coaching and goal-setting sessions to the hospital manager allows for specifically tailored performance planning with staff members. Acquiring the skills and knowledge to meet practice goals must be mentored by the manager and/or administrator; they are the ones accountable for augmenting the group's efforts with new resources from within.

- *Inventory management.* This will be one of the professional aspects of every hospital manager's job. It is estimated that one in five of all employees will likely "borrow" from the practice at some time without permission. This inventory management role will add both internal control and cost effectiveness items to the group administrator's development plan for inventory and fiscal accountability at each facility.

- *Practice personality.* Body language, phone communications, client relations, and intrastaff relationships need to convey concerned care, patient advocacy, and continuity of care. The hospital manager should be responsible for the smile and fun efforts; it will permeate the practice philosophy.

Routine bookkeeping, accounts receivable, billing, chart of accounts, problem-oriented medical record (POMR) quality assurance, and a host of other functions stand ready to be transferred once the hospital manager earns team trust and respect. Do not overwhelm a new manager with a job description and a pointing finger. The job is complex, and the training needed is a repetitive step-by-step procedure. One description will never suffice to explain the multiple interrelationships of a veterinary practice. Be patient and have fun.

Remember there are many styles of leadership (i.e., situational leadership, from autocratic to democratic and many points in between), and they need to be used like a scalpel, not a club. The staff is there because they care: we *train* dogs, but we *nurture* people. The uncommon leader develops people through work; the traditional manager only gets work done through people. The cute leadership phrases have deep meaning to the uncommon leader, and when you hire a practice manager or hospital administrator you have a choice: either develop and nurture the new administrator, allowing others to grow the practice for you, or train to process and stagnate your practice development. The choice is yours, and those surviving into the new millennium will know which choice to make!

MANAGEMENT EFFECTIVENESS QUESTIONNAIRE

INSTRUCTIONS

You will find 63 descriptive questions that will help you assess your current understanding and knowledge of this management stuff. Be very thoughtful as you evaluate your approach to management, then rate the extent to which each sentence describes what you do (not hope to do; what you are doing now!).

Answer every statement. Place an X in the box beside each statement that best describes your situation. If you need to change your answer, simply draw a circle around the first X, then mark a new X in the other box. **There are only three choices: U = Usually/Always, S = Sometimes, R = Rarely/Never.**

SAMPLE

To what extent do you:

		U	S	R
7.	Ensure a continuity of care within the medical records and that **every** doctor complies.	❏	❏	✗
34.	Not overlap staff member assignments to prevent duplication of effort and useless competition? (This answer indicates the manager usually did that.)	✗	❏	❏

THE QUESTIONNAIRE

To what extent do you:

		U	S	R
1.	Practice persuasion and coaching in the development of middle managers **before** delegation?	❏	❏	❏
2.	Believe in open-book management, since staff knows the daily deposits yet seldom understands the overhead?	❏	❏	❏
3.	Let go of the profit and loss numbers and focus on the programs and procedure numbers.	❏	❏	❏
4.	Ensure a continuity of care within the medical records and that **every** doctor complies?	❏	❏	❏

		U	S	R

5. Require standardization between doctors for wellness and preventive medical standards of diagnostics, immunizations, and other testing expectations? ❏ ❏ ❏

6. Develop outpatient nursing staff and leverage your professional time per client? ❏ ❏ ❏

7. Believe that a trained hospital administrator can do all you do, except for hands-on patient care? ❏ ❏ ❏

8. Block out a quiet-time hour (on practice time), free from phone calls and other interruptions, for planning? ❏ ❏ ❏

9. Take enough time (5–20 percent) to think what needs to be accomplished or changed, and what needs to stop? ❏ ❏ ❏

10. Devote concentrated, uninterrupted time to a single major problem? ❏ ❏ ❏

11. Concentrate on core value applications to important issues rather than just reacting to crises? ❏ ❏ ❏

12. Look for recurring crises to find system errors and correct them? ❏ ❏ ❏

13. Enforce meeting management, or if not in charge of meeting, indicate meeting management is needed? ❏ ❏ ❏

14. Regularly say "no" to those who want to do work which does not contribute to the success of the practice? ❏ ❏ ❏

15. Focus on needs for now and the future rather than just fixing antiquated systems or blaming others? ❏ ❏ ❏

16. Focus on the need to examine current priorities and recalibrate them to the community as required? ❏ ❏ ❏

	U	S	R

17. Remain flexible to change, yet successfully protect practice standards and priorities by refusing to do unnecessary things others want you to do? ❏ ❏ ❏

18. Regularly recommend reducing or eliminating programs, policy, or clutter that detracts from practice efficiency, staff effectiveness, or practice harmony? ❏ ❏ ❏

19. Keep your people involved on tasks that will provide a maximum impact on quality health care and client satisfactions? ❏ ❏ ❏

20. Limit your people's priorities to two or three items rather than constantly bombarding them? ❏ ❏ ❏

21. Courageously establish priorities (what is significant versus what is easy; what you believe is required versus what everyone else does)? ❏ ❏ ❏

22. Concentrate on staff members' strengths and build on them rather than worry about what they can't do? ❏ ❏ ❏

23. Overlook or forgive staff members' imperfect behavior that doesn't adversely affect their work or the practice? ❏ ❏ ❏

24. Place people in jobs that require them to grow, rather than in static positions, then give them new job demands when they are ready? ❏ ❏ ❏

25. Empower your staff members so you are free to concentrate on clients and patients? ❏ ❏ ❏

26. Expect your staff to get the right things accomplished, rather than just be busy? ❏ ❏ ❏

27. Challenge any policy, procedure, or other limitation which prevents your staff from being developed and utilized to their fullest potential? ❏ ❏ ❏

28. Assign yourself the most difficult tasks, then accomplish at least one significant item daily? ❏ ❏ ❏

		U	S	R
29.	Exercise good communication skills to achieve actions?	❏	❏	❏
30.	Give staff members your undivided time and attention when they need to discuss their concerns with you?	❏	❏	❏
31.	Share your feelings both as a person and as the boss to establish honest, open communication?	❏	❏	❏
32.	Each day provide feedback so others know how they are doing?	❏	❏	❏
33.	Provide immediate, yet face-saving, private reprimands when needed so staff members are aware of deviations from appropriate performance expectations?	❏	❏	❏
34.	Ask the staff clarifying questions. Then ask for their personal recommendations, rather than giving them the answers?	❏	❏	❏
35.	Not overlap staff assignments to prevent duplication of effort and useless competition?	❏	❏	❏
36.	Co-establish staff work agendas to blend practice objectives with your own improvement programs?	❏	❏	❏
37.	Review each staff member's approved performance plan (quarterly objectives for improvement) with middle managers, then adjust the objectives based on staff members' feedback on frustrations and internal road blocks?	❏	❏	❏
38.	Blend staff members' work needs and practice goals?	❏	❏	❏
39.	Assign projects completely by setting priorities, specifying tasks to be done and identifying measurable standards, setting progress review and completion dates, defining level of authority, and getting staff members' commitment to the project before assigning time line(s)?	❏	❏	❏

		U	**S**	**R**

| 40. | Keep your staff informed of vision or mission changes (problems, needs, objectives)? | ❑ | ❑ | ❑ |

| 41. | Identify and eliminate roadblocks to staff's performance as well as provide practice culture and logistical support? | ❑ | ❑ | ❑ |

| 42. | Periodically share performance information with staff so they will know how well they're meeting their objectives and how you feel about their work? | ❑ | ❑ | ❑ |

| 43. | Make logical and rational decisions based on facts. Then apply your gut feelings to reach a conclusion? | ❑ | ❑ | ❑ |

| 44. | Give decision-making authority and responsibility to the staff, including commitment of resources and the possibility of making mistakes? | ❑ | ❑ | ❑ |

| 45. | Lead a brainstorm session to solve problems rather than risk error by a yes/no answer of a single recommendation? | ❑ | ❑ | ❑ |

| 46. | Apply the experience and wisdom of others who are closest to the problem? Trust in the staff's opinion? | ❑ | ❑ | ❑ |

| 47. | Delegate responsibilities to trained and trusted staff members and refuse to make any decisions they should be making based on their training? | ❑ | ❑ | ❑ |

| 48. | Encourage your staff to be risk takers rather than evaders of failure who feel they have to check first with you on everything? | ❑ | ❑ | ❑ |

| 49. | Make quick decisions to keep the practice moving, but move slowly on those decisions that are harder to reverse or require major change efforts by team members? | ❑ | ❑ | ❑ |

| 50. | Practice a personally healthy lifestyle? | ❑ | ❑ | ❑ |

| 51. | Pursue your own ongoing business growth and development through reading, formal classroom work, on-the-job-learning, and understudying mentors? | ❑ | ❑ | ❑ |

		U	S	R
52.	Establish yourself as a crucial subordinate or mentor to the practice management team, to further your own release from practice management projects and allow you to develop additional career or avocational interests?	❑	❑	❑
53.	Feel comfortable with others being the authority figures and understand the middle manager's and the team's needs?	❑	❑	❑
54.	Invest time and effort to train practice staff members, including grooming someone to replace you in the future?	❑	❑	❑
55.	Handle conflicts assertively rather than passively-aggressively to rebuild bridges between the conflicting staff members?	❑	❑	❑
56.	Analyze any practice or personal failures, face the facts, decide future action, and bounce back?	❑	❑	❑
57.	Concentrate your efforts and the staff's efforts on significant areas of contribution and not on trivial, meaningless tasks?	❑	❑	❑
58.	Survey clients' perceptions of the practice and incorporate that information to meet clients' needs?	❑	❑	❑
59.	Evaluate the process for business and healthcare reasons rather than just because it's always been done that way?	❑	❑	❑
60.	Encourage staff brainstorming and innovation?	❑	❑	❑
61.	Increase productivity through better technology, staff training, performance planning with measurements, and continuously improving work systems.	❑	❑	❑
62.	Develop team building, fair treatment for staff, and socialization, and emphasize quality of work life?	❑	❑	❑
63.	Make the pursuit of excellence and high standards of job performance mission focus requirements?	❑	❑	❑

SCORING THIS ASSESSMENT

There are actually nine categories in the above 63 scenarios. There were not any right or wrong answers, there was only a statement of current situation; each practice is different, so the applications are different. The scoring is simple math, U = 5, S = 3, R = 1, for each question. So place the scores below:

Questions	Category System	
1–7	Healthcare Leadership	=
8–14	Time Management	=
15–21	Future Priorities	=
22–28	Build on Strengths	=
29–35	Personal Relationships	=
36–42	Outcome Management	=
43–49	Action Planning	=
50–56	Personal Development	=
57–63	Commitment Focus	=

Look at the totals on the right, ranging from 7 to 35 points in each category. Those categories with low numbers are potential areas for development and training by the hospital manager and practice leadership. Those categories with high numbers are potential areas for immediate delegation efforts, since the skills to train others are already there. This is a unique perspective for most veterinarians and practice managers, but it has proven very successful in other healthcare delivery settings. Try it. Test it for 90 days; you may just like it.

5 The Rest of the Story

Any time you think the problem is "out there,"
that very thought is the problem.
—Stephen R. Covey

Changing Attitudes

Focus on the Short Term

You are looking for management assistance, or you want to make a transition in your management style to a more productive format; that is why you are at Chapter Five in this book. The recent Leaders Conference, hosted by the American College of Healthcare Executives (ACHE), for CEOs of healthcare organizations, asked some targeted leadership questions of the participants. The ACHE wanted to help those already successful in the healthcare industry to share their perceptions with those looking to change the future for their organizations.

First, and most surprising, was that becoming the CEO of a hospital or an HMO was no longer seen as a definition of career success. Human health care and managed care present too many options for a position to define success. There was also a strong consensus that most young workers don't want to make long-term commitments (and this is something we also currently see in veterinary medicine). In fact, one human resource placement person stated, "The short term is very short, and there is no long term. We hire in the eternal present!" Practice owners, please take note. This focus on the short term is true not just of new veterinary medical graduates or new technicians; this attitude is the result of a generational evolution. Balanced lives are important and **must** be assertively addressed as we enter the new millennium.

New graduates, with degrees in business management or healthcare administration, no longer have management as a desirable end-career goal. Many of the highly school-trained, entry level middle managers want specialist roles, such as consulting, strategic planning, or even

marketing. It is an explosion of reality hitting the marketplace: workers are putting lifestyle **before** work ethics. Institutional leaders must
be mentors and nurturing partners with these entry level members of
the management team; the new talent has what is being called *negotiated commitment*. The best and brightest of these workers have already produced the following changes in the healthcare environment:

- Job sharing

- Causal business dress

- Telecommunicating

- Flex-time

- Self-governance

- Training provided as a term of hiring

- Limited, carefully defined, personal commitment

- Counteroffers rather than annual reviews

The days of expecting total commitment to a role or an employer are
over. The question most often asked of leaders in health care today, by
the new generation of managers and administrators in health care delivery environments, is, "How can I find a job that's useful, satisfying,
and rewarding, but not all-consuming?" In fact, the lifestyle-first attitude is so widespread in human health care now that it has lost its
shock value within human resource promotions. Veterinary medicine
practice owners, however, are still being shocked by this attitude.

Redefining Success

When the healthcare leaders were asked by ACHE to list three adjectives which best defined their career success, the answers included
such descriptive words as *respected, balanced, committed, ethical, innovative, focused, challenged, creative,* and *competent*. But these were
not the top five responses. The top five adjectives that defined career
success in their minds were *flexible* (45 percent), *visionary* (28 percent), *honest* (18 percent), *confident* (13 percent), and *energized* (10
percent).

To better understand these perceptions, conference organizers asked
the leaders what their top three career concerns were. In this case, responses were again varied, but the choices were far more limited in

scope. These responses included *job satisfaction* (31 percent), *achieving career goals* (26 percent), *acquiring new skills* (24 percent), *job security* (12 percent), *managing stress* (6 percent), and *other* (1 percent).

When asked if their definition of success was different today from when they entered the healthcare field, 68 percent said, "yes." Some of the most common ways the definition of success had changed included:

- *Degree of balance in their lives.* Define clearly what leaving before 6 p.m. and having work-free weekends really will cost the healthcare organization. Younger workers don't talk of money, power, and position; they talk of relationships and lifestyle needs. Money no longer feeds the monkey.

- *Possessing transferable skills.* Growth, not movement up the ladder, is important for self-esteem; new skills are more important than titles and salaries. The new generation can be lured by the siren song of new skills, and *routine work* is an obscenity that scares them away.

- *Their ability to adjust to changes in the field.* Strategic responses have replaced strategic planning; those in the outside world no longer will dance to the music determined to be best for them by the institution. Instead, the skilled leader watches the community and environmental trends and grabs opportunity as it flies by.

- *The degree of satisfaction they derived from their work.* No one in health care is a generalist anymore; everyone has a niche, and those in a niche that fulfills a viable passion will be inspired to excel. There is no success in passivity, even if it is competent, results-oriented passivity. The thrill of the job is replacing the lure of the retirement benefit package which kept the last generation hooked to the healthcare wagon.

- *The effect they have on their communities.* Making a difference in the lives of others is why many people enter health care and why almost everyone I know entered veterinary medicine. Social psychology is as important a course for leadership success as basic bookkeeping. The community in which the leader lives is part of the nurturing environment that makes the healthcare organization prosper or die. Good leaders feed community needs, so the community will feed the organization's needs.

Can you—the veterinary-interested reader—see how you make a difference? Today, more people in health care call themselves successful, at all levels of income and responsibility, because they make a difference in the lives of others. People enter veterinary medicine because it allows them to positively impact the health status of lesser animals, and some even do it because of the positive impact on the producer, the family, or the community. Others are interested in the way veterinary health care is being delivered, either because they want to increase access to veterinary medical care or because they think they can improve the quality of care. For people in health care today, making a difference will mean changing as needed to meet the changing needs of the clients, the community, and the staff.

Making Changes

Need for Leadership

There will always be traditionalists in veterinary medicine. There will always be veterinarians who will do whatever it takes to make their practice appear viable (maybe that is why there is such a high divorce rate in our profession). The number of these traditionalists is declining, however, because the values required to succeed in the past are no longer fashionable, or even relevant, in some communities. What is very clear is that today there are as many models for success as there are leaders in veterinary medicine. Right now, no one model dominates and no one leadership style can fit all occasions. The uncommon leader is needed in each practice, yet less than 10 percent of practices have true leadership. Management skills will be needed by the leadership of tomorrow, but more importantly, the managers of today must become the leaders of tomorrow. Those unwilling or unable to become leaders will need to become followers, or they will become obsolete in veterinary medicine and their community.

Resistance to Change

Seven thousand people died in one year in New York state as a result of negligent care; 99,000 patients were injured as a result of their medical care.
—Recent ACHE seminar

We all know that the healthcare systems in America are the best in the world. Community hospitals have followed the lead of business in an attempt to improve their systems. In this process, they have tried many approaches: *quality circles* did not work; *participative management* did not work; now *total quality management* (TQM) implemented as *continuous quality improvement* (CQI) is not working. It is traditional corporate culture, not the concepts, that have caused problems. One of the recent winners of the Baldridge Award for quality, Florida Power and Light, was heralded as a TQM winner. Within two years of winning the Baldridge Award, the CEO was fired due to the highest utility rates in the area and very unhappy employees. It seems that the Baldridge Committee considered Florida Power and Light's process, but not its outcomes. This almost sounds like a prototype for the average veterinary practice that is looking to solve all its problems by hiring a qualified practice manager or administrator. The culture of the veterinary practice was established by the leadership of the practice, which means changes must occur within the key players, hospital director, and practice owner(s) to allow the newly hired and well-qualified manager or administrator the latitude to build a better organization.

In a *USA Today* editorial (December 15, 1991), "The Tale of Health Care Could Induce Nausea," our clients were informed of the failings in healthcare delivery. This story, in many formats, has been repeated over and over at the end of the century because no one is making changes. In 1998, HCA Columbia crashed from a top 10 position in healthcare industry stocks to the very bottom of the list, due to a lack of ethical performance standards (and the subsequent litigation highlighting their shortfalls). Informed clients are more likely to return to a veterinary practice that delivers value within ethical limits. They are also more likely to leave a practice that charges for more than what the client *perceived* was received (this behavior is also called *unethical* if the communications were very poor). Some people quote the leading management articles or seminar courses as if the words were religious maxims; these words, however, seldom address the bioethical issues, personal relationships, or core values needed to maintain the social contract of healthcare delivery. Management and religion have a different orientation. Knowledge is not a single set of concepts.

The secret of business management, regardless of the premise or system, is to *get things done*. Look at the car industry. The Saturn took five years to come into the market, but the Lexus took only 13 months. The system that comes into the marketplace first has the advantage, if clients can differentiate between the products/providers. Savin identified the small copier market as an emerging need then took that business away from Xerox. While Savin rested on their accomplishments, Canon took the individual copier market lead from them. Last decade, we saw that Chrysler was in the financial hole, and everyone in their system knew they had to change; General Motors was $60 billion ahead and comfortable in their successful programs. Total quality management (TQM) was offered and accepted by both companies. Chrysler changed and Lee Iacocca became a legend. General Motors fired Ross Perot and has just posted the greatest loss in automotive history.

As we say in continuous quality improvement (CQI), when *pride* is the input, then *quality* will be the output clients perceive. When you establish a quality management program in any veterinary practice, the leadership often subconsciously prevents change. Change is critical for improvement; almost everyone agrees with this concept. On the other hand, most veterinarians resist operational changes. Operational signs that signal an environment where the management system myth has been so entrenched that it hinders the pride-quality relationship include the following:

- Slow implementation—extended time frames

- Little early business results for new ideas

- Data, studies, pilot programs, and go slow signals abound

- Passive resistance from old-timers (this-too-shall-pass attitude)

- Lack of buy-in and ownership by the staff

- The gimmick-based system is not self-sustaining

When detected, in part or together, the half-dozen signs listed above indicate that a myth has been implemented. Old habits are not allowing change to occur, so implementation efforts are impotent. Training the leadership helps, but training alone does not create results; commitment does. For example, it you want to improve the leadership and client-centered concern in your practice team, redesign your evaluation system for merit pay increases: tenure is not a reason for pay increases, and neither is popularity. (If you can't measure it, you can't manage it, right?) Then reexamine the systems that have been established for all pay increases in the practice, including the boss's pay. Merit pay increases should come from two sources: (1) 50 percent from a staff harmony evaluation and (2) 50 percent from a client return rate evaluation.

These are scary concepts, I know, and tough to implement, but the results are proven. If you believe in leadership rather than management, in outcomes rather than process controls, and in client satisfaction above policies, then you pursue *doing the right things* rather than *doing things right*. And you can accept, even encourage, the change process.

Are You Ready for Change?

A veterinary practice must be ready to accept change if it pursues total quality management (TQM) or continuous quality improvement (CQI). There is a formula for change (C), in which *dissatisfaction/discomfort desire to change* (D), the *participative process* needed to move to the new systems (P), and the *model* that can be accepted by all as a better world (M) each play an equal part.

$$C = D \times P \times M > \text{Cost}$$

If you remember high school math, you can see that if any one of these three formula elements becomes minimized, change does not readily occur. Note that a successful change outcome must make more money than it costs to produce it. There are three areas to evaluate if you are considering proactive change:

- Lack of organizational change readiness:
    - ✓ Imbalance between flexibility and control.
    - ✓ History of repeated failure of new programs.
    - ✓ Notable for management bandaids and patches.
    - ✓ Crisis reactive in lieu of vision proactive.

- Violation of proper change sequence:
    - ✓ High human resources turnover rates mean staff disbelief.
    - ✓ Proper change sequence—first mission, structure, and accountability, then rewards.
    - ✓ Greater priorities—turnover decimation, client servicing, competitive and financial survival.

- Poor support of implementation systems:
    - ✓ Dollars strangling the recommended solutions.
    - ✓ Lack of desire-for-change leadership and follow-through.
    - ✓ Dysfunctional organizations kill their young.

Inept change management is often based on new buzz phrases rather than detailed understandings. Great ideas are seen as magic bullets, and the programs are tried in isolation. There are even some "leaders" who force their new insights on others in the organization and short-circuit the team change process. There are many who initiate extensive training programs that target competence but rarely change the coordination requirements to allow proactive change. The practice culture must be ready to change, and the staff must really believe that a total overhaul is needed. Commitment to excellence and competency requires time and effort, and the quick-fix gimmicks of the past do not belong in the future of veterinary practice management.

Critical Practice Tools

Performance Planning

Those who have used supervisory performance plans in lieu of traditional appraisal scoring know that they involve a quarterly process of making changes and improving knowledge/skill abilities. The experience of Veterinary Practice Consultants® shows that we can teach the principles and ensure that the practice owners and managers understand the concept of key result areas (KRAs), but all too often, the practice does not have the discipline to make it happen every quarter. In the simplest terms, performance planning is a joint process of setting 90-day goals in seven areas of expected outcomes: client satisfaction, quality, personal growth, organizational climate, innovation, productivity, and economics. Many practices are willing to talk about change, but setting quarterly change goals is uncomfortable for them; they would rather revert than change. The reality is far different for those that make the commitment and have the discipline to use assertive planning; when the key result areas (KRAs) are combined with the concepts of CQI, five concept areas need to be monitored for measurement of success:

- Get the right things done, **now**.

- Continuous quality improvement is action, not a study of data accumulation.

- Increase revolutionary change gangs, SWOT [strength and weakness (inside)/opportunity and threats (outside)] teams, hot idea teams (HITs), do it groups (DIGs), etc.

- The leader manages the *why* and watches out for the people.

- There is constant dynamic interaction between the KRAs.

True leaders understand the importance of their people. When starting the morning briefings during Desert Storm, the key question by the general was, "What have you done for the troops today?" At one hospital, client service is simply defined as causing "Wow!" perceptions in clients. At Hyatt, they learned that if they made people feel at home, they couldn't charge for the special services people want when away from home; they had to do more. The planning and commitment choice is yours, but a team approach is far more fun that the traditional I-will-do-it-all approach.

Forming Alliances

Someone once said, "It is lonely at the top,"
but the fact is it can be lonely anywhere in
the organization.
—Dr. T.E. Catanzaro

Veterinary medicine is a lonely business for most veterinarians. The doctor is always surrounded by people looking for answers: staff, clients, and the community. The owner is afraid to talk to other practices, sometimes because of the Federal Trade Commission (FTC) threats about fee sharing or restraint of trade issues, often because they are perceived as competitors by their colleagues, but most often because veterinarians believe they can do everything themselves—**always**. The need for those in small businesses (that is the banker's definition of most veterinary practices) to ally with others is complex and multifaceted. Most practitioners need at least three primary alliances: one alliance to exchange information, one to accomplish major community or environmental issues, and one to relax. As veterinary medicine enters the new millennium, the need for collegiality has never been greater, from increasing community involvement, to more personal association support, to the use of NOAH or VIN computer linkages, to the need to refer cases to colleagues who have specialized equipment and/or training.

This triple alliance structure also applies to the practice manager, hospital administrator, and even the group administrator. Alliances and interactions within the community are essential for their effectiveness. In the board certification with ACHE, I must retest (oral and written in the 10 areas shown in the Appendix B) every five years, but I do not even qualify for reexamination unless I am active in some community activity. I have always been involved in the youth programs in any community in which I reside, generally through the Boy Scout movement, but ACHE diplomate candidates may choose their church, Rotary, Optimists, Lions, or a host of other civic organizations. It does not matter, just choose and move. Encouraging these alliances means giving the veterinary hospital administrator the time for a Rotary breakfast or lunch, for early departure for evening church functions, for a liberally free weekend if he/she is doing Scout outings, and concurrently, for some daytime latitude to coordinate these community activities. This is all part of small business, of developing a well-rounded manager, and it sure helps the practice stay in touch with community trends and desires.

The isolation veterinarians make for themselves is a manifestation of our professional belief that we *must* perform. In many smaller practices, which have been built by the sweat of a single visionary veterinarian, this attitude has been passed on to the key players (at least to those who have survived the stress and pressure of learning the demanding doc-controls-everything environment). Every member of the veterinary healthcare delivery team has this dedication to performance; although exceptions exist, they are so few that addressing them is not worth the required management effort. In large practices with multiple full-time doctor environments, it is more likely that client-centered, patient-advocative dedication and commitment will be present in the animal caretakers, technician nurses, receptionist team, associate veterinarians, and even significant others. The leaders who built the practice, however, are often stressed with requirements beyond their experience and comfort zone. The drive to be all you can be and an I-can-do-it-myself attitude often isolate each person from those who care or who could help.

Building Pride

FACT People must be able to meet or exceed a standard measure of expectations to have pride in what they do.

As a builder of practices, a consultant for those who want to be more than they are, I have seen the full spectrum of personal commitment. Sure, some people look for personal wealth at the expense of others, but most veterinarians I have met measure themselves and their practices against an inner yardstick of worth, and their personal pride is the driving force toward the search for excellence. Concurrently, most practice managers I have met measure themselves and their performance against the owner's yardstick of worth. As a motivation for excellence, the personal pride of CVPMs and credentialed hospital administrators must be allowed to surface as they take ownership of their jobs. The hot button for the individual staff member is generally different than the driving force of the manager, administrator, or owner. Mission focus means moving toward a higher level of healthcare delivery excellence; it is the application of core values to every element of the practice operations. The paraprofessionals within a practice are dedicated and, most often, underpaid, which reflects their true dedication to the profession, the clients, and the patients.

The challenge for a consultant is to find out what measurements (values) have been engraved onto the specific practice's or veterinarian's inner yardstick. The same yardstick problem exists within any community of veterinarians (with or without an association). The fact is, in most every case the values and measurements are not engraved, written, or even espoused; they are like shifting sands, and everyone must guess what is expected. While I was with the American Animal Hospital Association, the question was phrased, "Are we an association of companion animal hospitals, do we represent practice owners, are we guardians of the cutting edge of companion animal healthcare delivery, or do we represent all our members?" If the standard measures are not well defined, and if they are not built on the organization's inviolate core values, then expectations cannot be exceeded by anyone on the team. Only by providing an environment and culture that allows the staff to exceed expectations can we grow personal pride; clients perceive pride as quality, and that is the cutting edge in client perceptions of healthcare delivery!

Pride is essential in a service industry and critical in the healthcare profession; clients equate pride in performance with quality. It is their only measurement. External pride in the veterinary profession is eroded by isolationism and competition: fear of the diminishing dollar reduces the search for an effective alliance, for an exchange of needs, and for assisting each other. Consider the internal practice situation where competency measures are developed by the staff as a response to some inaccurate perception of what "they" think. Lack of communication is a barrier to success, and the inaccurate competency measures can produce a significant breakdown of pride because it is very difficult for someone to work toward nonexistent measurements.

Uncertainty and misperceptions in this situation arise from isolation and poor communication within the practice. The same principle exists between practices and between colleagues. Do not respond to inaccurate perceptions of what "they" think; instead, reach out, telephone, even go to the other practitioner and discuss the issue(s). You may even find an ally.

The Present Is Rooted in the Past

Most business executives recognize the leadership of the Harvard Business School in the management trends of the United States. What is most interesting is the realization that the leaders of the 1990s and new millennium graduated in the 1970–1980 time frame (not unlike the owners of the multi-doctor veterinary practices). If we look at the selection criteria for Harvard for the Class of 1970 (*Business Week*, June 18, 1990), we see why American business trends at the turn of this century are as they are. We can learn from this insight and apply some of the factors to the trends seen in veterinary practices today.

Anthony G. Athos was the admissions director and professor of organizational behavior for the 742 future leaders of the Class of 1970. Phrases he used to describe the selection criteria for the future leaders that Harvard Business School sought to educate during those years included the following:

- "They were not elegant sheep."

- "We looked for people who stirred the pot rather than guarded it."

- "To foster debate in the classroom, students were divided into sections that were likely to clash."

- "The Harvard Business School is designed to teach the student to make quick decisions, establish priorities, and handle mind-numbing pressure."

- "These will be the movers and shakers, the builders and turnaround artists, the deal makers and green mailers."

- "The case study competition was a tiger pit, there was always the threat of being eaten; in the first year, students could do nothing good and in the second year, they could do no wrong."

- "The Harvard Business School approach was a competitive envi-

ronment that was a 'mind-forming' rather than 'knowledge-form-
ing' experience."

As compared to the all-male class of 1949 (the group that formed
the business trends seen in 1970), the class of 1970 centered on diversity: 31 women, 25 blacks, state school recruits, and even military
academy students. Although they were the most diverse class ever en-
rolled at the Harvard Business School, they remained comparatively
conservative. When the Harvard students voted to strike in 1969, only
the schools of business and law remained open. This was a class with
a purpose, and they knew what they wanted.

This is the class that produced Ellen Marram, CEO of Nabisco, one
of the highest ranking women in corporate America; and Robert Ryan,
CFO of Union Texas Petroleum, one of the few blacks in senior management at a public corporation. The interesting factor is that the majority of the CEOs in the class (only 93 of 723 work in *Business Week
1000* companies and only 26 rate a listing in *Who's Who in Finance
and Industry*) have distinguished themselves as entrepreneurs and
small-business people. They value job satisfaction and independence
more highly than they do the salary of a corporate giant.

From that generation's loins come the veterinary students of today,
those who want a maximum 40-hour work week commitment, no
weekend or evening on-call, and a salary that allows pursuit of outside
activities (just like their parents have). These students were raised in a
what's-in-it-for-me environment, a very lonely atmosphere for a
teenager. In many cases, these dedicated young doctors **never** saw the
dues their families paid to get where the family or parents were when
their own memories started. If these concepts are accepted, then the
lack of alliances, the reduced association support, and the reluctance
to refer are understandable. Understandable does not make it right, but
it does mean that an uncommon leader is needed to change the trends
in the new millennium.

Expectations

FACT

Expectations must be realistic and practical, and there must be a willingness to "break the bond" if they "don't cut the mustard."

In the practice setting, every veterinary practice owner knows he/she
must be ready to clearly state practice philosophy and set standards in

clear and concise terms. Unfortunately, the statement of philosophy is usually asked for in times of conflict and stress, and situational responses abound. The identification of core values and inviolate leadership-driven beliefs, and the the establishment of a clear mission focus, for consistent application, will mark the successful veterinary practice of the new millennium. In associations, which are, by contrast, usually based on public relations and volunteers, clarity is lost when current elected officers try to be all things for all people (*politics*), and expectations in associations are further blurred by membership diversification and the traditional committee compromise and consensus systems. A veterinary practice must have a clear mission focus so that clear and consistent expectations can be created. When a veterinary practitioner decides to refer a client/patient to another veterinarian, sharing expectations makes the referral (a working alliance) less risky. Clear expectations facilitate smoother relationships not only within the practice but also between practices (so that good working alliances can be formed). Clear expectations also allow staff to excel and thereby create pride in the staff and a perception of quality in practice clients.

Patient Advocacy

> **FACT** Clients will perceive patient advocacy as caring, the caring as pride in healthcare delivery; and the pride as quality excellence.

From this end-of-century generation also comes the better client, the upper middle class pet owner, age 35 to 55, with discretionary dollars to spend. These clients look for veterinary health care that matches their value system: highly organized, based on facts and professionally sound decisions, and oriented to outcome. The studies show that about 75 percent of the top-end clients would prefer to be sent to a specialist for resolution. This is the group that can be swayed to a well-stated cause, by the public relations effort of a local professional association or by a practitioner who clearly states the pet's need then offers two ways to say "yes" to the client.

The high technology diagnostics available to our profession, and our clients, are increasing daily, but the delivery of these new services must be client-centered and value-based, and staff delivering these services must exhibit a high level of personal regard for the role of patient advocate. This group of 35- to 55-year-old pet owners readily understands the patient advocate approach of the progressive veterinary practice. This is, after all, the generation that demonstrated in the streets of Cambridge, at Kent State, and on college campuses across the nation. To attract and keep these clients, the practice must create in them a perception of excellence.

This perception of excellence is created by the pride in their work shown by all staff members, from doctors to animal caretakers. This pride will show in a myriad of ways, from a well-organized (not cluttered) front desk, to clean facilities (no strong disinfectant odors or animal waste odors), to prompt attention to the needs and concerns of clients. Staff who take pride in their performance and work as advocates for the patient will create a perception of excellence in clients which will help attract and hold them to the practice.

Average Is Not Enough

The trends of the new millennium are performance excellence in companion animal and equine healthcare delivery and economic excellence in production animal health care. Gone are the days of being adequate. Veterinarians are no longer seen as being in short supply or as a valued asset to attract to the community with incentives; poor distribution does exist, but that is another issue for this profession in the new millennium. Banks now want at least 20–30 percent down to start a new practice in town, if you can prove you don't need the capital. The need to consolidate inpatient care services at fewer facilities has become a critical economic necessity.

No longer can we expect a purely client-centered approach to overcome a competition-centered approach in the quest for new clients. Networking between practices makes the community client pie a shared resource of opportunity rather than the object of a tug-of-war between colleagues. The client-centered approach can help bond the client to the practice and possibly increase return visits, but mobile America requires a constant infusion of new ideas and new modalities to make veterinary health care seem unique. Clients are needed to keep any veterinary practice healthy (10 percent of all transactions should be new clients), and an alliance is needed to keep the community group of veterinary practice healthy. The Strategic Assessment Tools in Appendix E provides a format for making these evaluations, but do not replace the colleague outreach that has been waning in our profession.

Organize to Capitalize

FACT When it's lonely at the top, you are forgetting to talk with the people at the bottom!

How an association or a practice organizes to meet these new demands indicates how well the leadership has assessed the competitive environment. It will take the perceived quality associated with an organized and dedicated professional healthcare delivery team to differentiate the practice and this profession in the competitive veterinary marketplace. It is the client's perception that will differentiate the practice, and the practice that differentiates itself from the graduates of the Harvard Business School Class of 1970 will be seen as the progressive leader in the veterinary medical healthcare delivery community. This means the isolated veterinary practice owner who tries to make all the management decisions from the top becomes an obstacle to success.

Using the staff to achieve practice goals is the secret we most often discuss and share; our consulting business is teaching practice owners how to build on staff strengths and community opportunities. Inversely, the demands that a hospital director puts on the practice team, such as percentage growth goals, are too often taken for granted as appropriate; staff cannot affect percentages, but they can affect clients, patient healthcare delivery, and in some cases, the organizational climate of harmony. This lack of workable factors comes from the same indifference that practitioners show toward local and state associations, as well as other practices. We can no longer be islands of excellence, we must depend upon those around us for the alliance of progress. Yesterday's innovation is today's mediocrity.

As veterinarians, we usually ask those who work with us to meet our own high standards in the practice, in professional associations, and even at the referral practice. Seldom are staff members paid to perform at this level of intensity and dedication, but they do believe in us, and they attempt to perform at a higher level of productivity. Training is most often inadequate (recurring in-service training is seldom seen in veterinary practices, even though we have seen a doubling of knowledge within this profession in only two years). The average veterinary practice's leadership support of team development and community alliances is generally less than optimum, and the veterinarian's personal commitment waivers with time. This type of scenario concurrently prevents the team (association, practice, or colleague) from asking for help to cope with these productivity demands.

Caring Leadership: Individuals Count

 The importance of the individual, staff, or client, must remain a critical factor in every veterinary practice management plan.

The isolation a veterinarian creates by repeatedly asking for increased productivity from self and others can be mediated. Association exchanges or an alliance of practices provides a calibration to reality. This is the basic principle of the traditional "20 groups" seen at the end of the decade. Twenty similar practices (size and philosophy) share economic information via an accountant who compiles the data; establishes ranges, averages and medians; and redistributes the data back to the 20 practices. This sharing of information allows self-calibration. An association provides calibration, outside the practice, to the needs of the profession; and an alliance of practices provides healthcare delivery calibration to the expanding capabilities of the profession. The lack of support for local, state, and national associations stems from the introspective perspective of the potential membership, not from the elected officers and committee members of the association. An association's success mimics the alliance of practices within the catchment community; weak associations reflect weak professional alliances.

In a changing veterinary practice, after the first set of productivity responses from the staff, the leadership needs to look elsewhere rather than asking more of the existing staff or themselves. When sharing the effort becomes necessary, the next step is to network within the professional association, with other community organizations, or with other veterinary facilities. The alternating internal effort and external effort will keep a balance in community support programs as well as in the scope of service offered by any specific practice. These alliance relationships will often bring to light people who are actually interesting as individuals, and these contacts may facilitate a social life away from practice. Veterinary practice needs to be fun to prevent burnout, and if fun does not come from within the practice, it must be developed outside.

Most people who work in the veterinary profession do so because of a compassion for animals and a commitment to the animals' welfare.

When the drive to success overshadows compassion, when expansion becomes more important than caring, it is time to reevaluate the pursuit of practice excellence in human resource terms.

If we don't consider each person's characteristics and needs, we can isolate our staff members within themselves and the team will suffer. Each person must be seen as a resource, and everyone realizes today that our valuable resources can be depleted. A good leader knows and uses his/her resources effectively (money, time, people, knowledge, clients, etc.). These resources include the strengths of the team members. Leadership skills can be learned, but this does not guarantee that a practice can implement the skills without help and continued reminders from outside sources. The practice, association, or veterinary medical leadership needs to reach out, to be sensitive, and to use individuals for their strengths without draining them of their individuality.

Continuous quality improvement requires every person to take pride in what he/she does every day. It means staff members have the right, the accountability, and the responsibility to make their day better, to make their jobs better, and to make the client feel better about the practice. In professional association work, it means to improve and strengthen the profession in the community. In a practice alliance, it means to expand the services available within the community while conserving capital by not duplicating equipment and specialty services. In practice consulting, it means tailoring the skill set to the practice's strengths, building a set of incremental steps for transition from where they are to where they want to be, and then mentoring the process step-by-step. The environment does not matter; we all need to practice continuous quality improvement in every relationship, whether it is personal, community, or business. If we are not attempting to make tomorrow better than today, or next week better than this week, then we are only holding on to yesterday, and yesterday will never get us into the new millennium.

This process requires translating the leadership of tasking into the ability to promote the assignment of accountabilities. It means asking questions before determining action within a sphere of influence. It means caring—caring about the quality of life of each individual, caring about the quality of care of the patients, and caring about the perceptions of those around us. Unless we care, and make the effort to listen, we will be alone in every crowd.

Creating and Controlling the Chaos of Change

We dance around in a ring and suppose,
But the secret sits in the middle and knows.
—Robert Frost

Mother Nature is one of the best teachers we have ever found, and we can learn from that gracious lady: she is in continuous change. Picture the hurricane. Pure chaos when viewed from the ground, it is a self-regulating, ebb and flow, continual process of rhythmic dynamics when pictured from the air. When north of the equator, hurricanes always rotate counterclockwise (just like water in the toilet bowl) and expend energy as they reach land: they are predictable. The DNA molecule is a similar flux and flex structure, seemingly completely unorganized until Watson and Crick told us what to look for when viewing the double helix. Then evolution started to become defined.

In our personal lives, as in nature, continuous change is required; this change can also be called *evolution*. In the business of healthcare delivery, evolution requires continuous quality improvement from each individual on the team. When the veterinary practice is viewed as a living, evolving organism, it makes sense for every component (person) to become involved.

Quantum Physics Replaces Mechanistic Process

Order and chaos are two forces and exist in relationship.
They are mirror images, one containing the other, a
continual process where a system can leap into chaos and
unpredictability, yet within that state be held within
parameters that are well-ordered and predictable.
—Margaret Wheatley
Leadership and the New Science

In the past decade of veterinary practice management, we have learned to build job descriptions, policy manuals, and "wire diagrams" to show the organization and structure of the practice. Somehow, these labors of management have helped very few practices prosper. As this decade ends and the next begins, we must disconnect from mechanistic views and make the transition to the fluid energy and force-field thinking of the current universe: we must accept chaos as a critical element of success.

Plato talked of the reality of perceptions as a man chained to a cave wall, facing the stone, unable to turn and see the rest of the cave. Plato said a giant fire in the center of the cave could be truth, reality, knowledge, the actual life force, but the poor man chained to the wall would only perceive the fire as shadows. Those shadows would be of his own reflection, but they would be his reality since the chains held him fast. Plato said men needed to turn 180 degrees to perceive the reality of life, but very few could since their chains of bias and prejudice were too tight. Creative chaos counters the destructive nature of stability and rigidity.

The core vision, values, and competencies of a practice prevent anarchy. Clarity of purpose increases staff buy-in. People are the true competitive advantage, and if their constraints are removed, they will stop reacting to chaos and cause it. In chaos, the true assets are ideas. Ideas fuel Plato's fire, the fire of reality. Strategic planning has proven to be ineffective, but then, look at the definition of evolution. Who has been able to predict the evolution of Mother Nature? Even McDonald's could not strategically predict the uproar caused by Styrofoam cartons, but they listened, changed, and saved money when they initiated the use of recycled paper.

There are three important elements in developing creative chaos:

1. Learning from the clients can be termed *strategic client response (SCR)* if action is taken within seven days of discovery. Clients are continually teaching, but many practices have quit learning. In most every community, the veterinary market does not exist anymore. A practice has one client at a time, and must ensure that each client returns. If a veterinary practice team centers on each client as if he/she is a special asset, the market share will take care of itself. In some practices where staff members really listen to clients, there will be occasional lighthouse clients. These clients are animal owners who cut through the fog and point the way for the future. They provide the early warning signs of evolution. The secret of success is how quickly the practice responds to client requests, rather than when the strategic plan is modified.

2. *Prime competitive advantage (PCA).* The staff is the prime competitive advantage (PCA) of a practice. A practice can either hire the best or hire warm bodies. When a practice hires the best, they must

be treated the best. The staff is the first and most important client of a veterinary practice; how you treat the staff will be reflected in how the staff treats the clients. Staff members must be given the freedom to make bold bets: implemented ideas can also be termed continuous quality improvement (CQI). The eleventh commandment (as developed by 3M) is simply, **never** kill an idea. If a practice counts ideas rather than paper towels; if the bookkeeper can tell you how many ideas were implemented rather than how many checks were written; and if the 90–90 rule is in effect (approve 90 percent of the ideas in seven days, and implement them within 90 days), then success is at hand.

3. *Uncommon leaders.* The practice must have business commandos, that is, leaders who are willing to be eccentrics, radicals, and gunfighters. Rubber Maid (the most admired business of 1994 according to *Fortune* magazine) has a corporate goal that one new product **must** be introduced each day of the year; in 1994, they introduced over 400 products. Their CEO, Wolfgang Schmidt, listens to trees, kids, trends, and clients, not accountants or conservatives; do you think anyone at Rubber Maid ever ignores any suggestion with this leadership standard in effect? What would happen if this occurred in veterinary practices?

The Renaissance Prescription

So, we watch Mother Nature, we accept quantum physics (we even know that light can be bent now), and we accept that the hottest selling car in America is the "cozy coupe" by Rubber Maid (500,000 units sold in 1994). We also know that plants are not enhanced by a single new gimmick being added; they routinely need water, sun, nutrients, pest protection, replanting, air, fertilization, carbon dioxide, and in some species, regular nurturing. Plants replicate by rhizomes, root systems, and miniaturization (seeds), and some even lose leaves as they grow. Veterinary practices work better when smaller teams replicate the vision and values of the practice and when nonproductive teams are allowed to be pruned.

The renaissance prescription, a specific **Rx** for success, has seven points:

1. **R**enew mission focus—commitment, challenge, passion for the cause.

2. **R**efocus business—client access, quality, cost-benefit, relationships.

3. **R**evitalize culture—effervescence, openness, new ideas, power-up innovation.

4. **R**ebirth leadership—samurai dedication, centurion loyalty, trust in people.

5. **R**ebuild the team—integrate, increase learning, beat 'em with brains, listen.

6. **R**eform the organization—lose dead weight, redesign jobs, set fewer boundaries.

7. **R**eengineer work systems—core value–based, lean and mean, meet challenges, solve problems.

Entering the New Playing Field

In 1987, Tom Peters wrote *Thriving on Chaos: Handbook for a Management Revolution,* and in 1989 Richardo Semelar wrote "Managing without Managers" in the *Harvard Business Review* (Sept-Oct 1989, 76–84). Yet we now see articles like "Changing the Role of Top Management: Beyond Structure to Processes" published in the *Harvard Business Review* (Jan-Feb 1995, 86–96), as if we didn't take the hint during the previous decade. The fact is, in veterinary medicine, super stores and public corporate practices are moving into the neighborhood because **no one** was willing to make the practice culture change to meet emerging client needs. The chaos created by this change in delivery modalities can be controlled, but not prevented, especially if practices are willing to cause their own chaos in their community's veterinary healthcare delivery systems.

The modern veterinary practice will be based on a triad formed by the healthcare provider, the staff, and the client (as queen or king). Trait labels such as competitive, robust, patient advocative, fast, dominant, flexible, adaptable, fun, innovative, and caring will be used to describe the winners. Pressures such as alternative providers, the knowledge explosion, litigation, resource scarcity, competitors, market changes, regulations, the cost of technology, and uncertainty will cause six key leadership areas to emerge as we enter the new millennium:

• *Client focus.* Easy access, rapid strategic client response (SCR), decreased costs, increased quality factors, removal of negatives, adding to value perceived, friendly facilities, greater market service, addressing wants and meeting needs.

- *Systems controlled.* Redesign jobs, reengineer functions, streamline cycle time, lead the benchmarks, brass tack tough adherence to values and vision, solid measurements for outcome expectations, and success celebrations.

- *Associate empowerment.* Hired doctors and staff unilaterally serve the client and improve the system, increase training and nurturing for individuals and teams, use the respect-recognition-responsibility formula, and increase utilization and freedom.

- *Uncommonly led.* Grow the prime competitive advantage with a positive client attitude (PCA^2), fit the organization to the users and doers, listen to clients and staff, believe in innovation and creativity, and get results and ideas rather than just status; just do it (JDI) becomes the requirement.

- *Values driven.* Core values are inviolate—effervescent culture and vision, kill problems rather than ideas, fun and celebration, bias for action and JDI, creative chaos, increase speed and adaptability, decrease barriers to change and innovation.

- *Mission focus.* Replace the words with applications that are repeated daily, using the above five factors, which are targeted on operations and personal relationships.

The real secret of empowerment is to get off the back of the staff: stop undermining the team. Take down the fences put up in the past, those caused by "Why did you do *that?*" questions and "We never did it that way!" statements. Put into place the B-HAGs (Big Hairy Audacious Goals). A "do it" project for any B-HAG has 30 days to get started and 90 days to get solved; warp speed is real in change management. If a problem solution cannot be initiated within 30 days, or resolved within 90 days, it **must be** redefined into smaller pieces that can be. The **minimum** idea goal for any veterinary practice which desires to excel in the new millennium needs to be one B-HAG for every staff member every quarter, with a 75 percent staff participation annually. In the first year of the process, the B-HAGs often need to be monthly staff meeting ideas, just so people will **believe** that change is a performance expectation. Staff participation needs to be over 75 percent when doing monthly staff meeting B-HAG programs; a fast scale-up for everyone is required for success.

The intellectual capital of a practice team is an intangible asset, but like a force field, it is real; having poor management systems does not mean there is no value in the practice team. In the series, *Star Trek, The Next Generation*, the captain is seldom out on point during strife; the phrase "Make it so!" stems from the team having the options, presenting the alternatives, and being trusted to implement their ideas. Many veterinary practice ideas have failed only because the hospital director or practice manager could not form the words, "Make it so!" In associations, the exact same stagnation issue is present; the group is afraid to trust someone or some committee and say, "Make it so!" This situation is not atypical, and veterinary medicine is not alone. Most business groups do not fully appreciate their teams and the ability of the team members to resolve issues without management's specific approval of the process: they do not respect the assets they have within their own ranks. Citibank has estimated their intellectual capital to be three to four times the book value of their business.

Remember Mother Nature? Look to her for the secrets of innovation and creativity. Human intelligence (HI) is not located in a specific part of the brain; it emerges with neural conversation, millions of messages expending energy to get a thought. If we expand the concept, then organizational intelligence (OI) would be the result of staff and client conversation. Who's got the brainpower?

It is not that a leader does not get great ideas, but a great leader lets the team members enhance the ideas until they become theirs. The leader of tomorrow creates the environment that nurtures change. The vision and values brought to bear by the veterinary leaders of tomorrow will be centered on client needs and rapid response to those needs (SCR). Great leaders cause conversation and feedback in this new open environment; they use all the brains available to resolve a problem (PCA). Change becomes the expectation (JDI), creative chaos is the standard used to measure innovation and creativity (OI), and together these elements become continuous quality improvement (CQI). Create chaos and you can control it; allow someone else to create it and you can only react to it. The choice is yours!

READY FOR CHANGE ASSESSMENT

Managing change is becoming more than an option; it is an increasingly critical element of practice survival. As such, change management is the defining trait of excellence for managers in the new millennium. The pace of change caused by new technology, competition, deregulation, community awareness, and other factors has made being a master of change necessary for the modern veterinary administrator. This assessment will help you gain a better idea of the approaches and strategies that can be pursued in order to be effective. The instrument will also help you create an action plan when you have to control chaos by causing change.

On the following pages you'll encounter 56 questions to help you assess your current knowledge of this exciting management subject. For each statement, you are asked whether you Agree (A) or Disagree (DA). If you feel ambivalent, choose the response that is closest to your primary feeling about the subject. Be sure to mark an answer by placing an X in the box beside each statement that most nearly describes how you feel. If you wish to change your answer, draw a circle around the first X and mark a new X in the other box.

Assessment

	Agree	Disagree
1. Knowledge is doubling every two years, making everybody's job obsolete.	❑	❑
2. Veterinarians can expect that the rate of change will stay about the same in private practice in the new millennium.	❑	❑
3. Change is caused primarily by practice leaders, new technology, and organized veterinary medicine groups.	❑	❑
4. The many positive changes that are being created in society make most people look forward to living in the future.	❑	❑
5. Most change is linear and evolutionary, not revolutionary with major breaks from the past.	❑	❑

	Agree	Disagree
6. Most practice managers make the greatest number of changes in their second and third year of occupying a position.	❏	❏
7. Change management is primarily technical problem solving, not people managing.	❏	❏
8. A manager should make his job different from what it was under his predecessor.	❏	❏
9. A manager's own willingness to change is essential in getting other staff members to accept changes.	❏	❏
10. Traditional practice managers are the biggest organizational obstacles to change, not doctors, resources, staff, or clients.	❏	❏
11. Innovation and creativity is a key result area for members of the management team to achieve through their people.	❏	❏
12. When the practice manager announces a change to the staff, he or she should retract it if it is not well received.	❏	❏
13. A change that isn't working should be tossed out and the old way reinstated.	❏	❏
14. Only a few staff members have any worthwhile ideas to improve the effectiveness of their practice.	❏	❏
15. After announcing a change decision, a manager receives more information that leads her/him to believe the change is a mistake. He/she should retract the decision and apologize for the error.	❏	❏
16. Suggestion box systems work well because the suggestion goes to a neutral party instead of to the person who has to implement it.	❏	❏
17. Money or prizes are necessary in order for staff to give a large number of ideas and suggestions.	❏	❏

	Agree	Disagree
18. Staff members who suggest changes should be encouraged to try them out.	❑	❑
19. Asking people for their ideas before a decision is made will not make them more receptive to the decision than those who weren't asked.	❑	❑
20. The manager's job is complicated by quality circles, or other relationships, which consume too much time for the small amount of productivity output they achieve.	❑	❑
21. Staff members, not their managers, should be seen as the source of most ideas concerning improvement of practice operations.	❑	❑
22. Getting people dissatisfied over the status quo or present method is a good idea in getting people to accept change.	❑	❑
23. Circulating reports of problems with the current systems is a good idea if you're contemplating changing.	❑	❑
24. Client evaluation of products/services is the best source for creating dissatisfaction energy to drive improvements.	❑	❑
25. Dissatisfaction over the present situation is more often a cause of change than the desire to improve the present situation, e.g., "negative" energy drives change more the "positive" desire.	❑	❑
26. Reports and measures have been found to be a major cause of energy changes in staff, by showing them the variance between their actual performance and the expected practice standards.	❑	❑
27. Making change requires an immense amount of energy from the administrator, middle managers and doctors: the number of major changes that any manager can successfully push through is limited.	❑	❑

	Agree	Disagree
28. When practice-wide apathy or inertia is present, usually little support can be found for change.	❏	❏
29. It's usually not a good idea to tell the staff members too far in advance about changes that will affect the practice.	❏	❏
30. Concerning change, it is usually better to communicate with a practice group than to talk to people individually.	❏	❏
31. Change should be discussed with the informal group leader(s) of the practice before trying to sell it to other staff members.	❏	❏
32. Taking people's feelings into account is more important than logical explanations about the change itself.	❏	❏
33. Change should never be implemented without an abundance of communication and staff participation.	❏	❏
34. Resistant subordinates should be tightly controlled so that others won't follow their example.	❏	❏
35. Communicating about the reasons for change is not necessary if the manager knows that people are going to resist anyway.	❏	❏
36. Once a practice-wide change is decided upon by the staff, it should be implemented immediately.	❏	❏
37. Unpopular changes should always proceed slowly in order to gain acceptance.	❏	❏
38. Changes leading to staff termination or realignment should have this element communicated before the change is implemented.	❏	❏
39. Change necessary for practice survival is accepted by most staff members.	❏	❏
40. Decisions to change should be based only on the facts.	❏	❏

	Agree	Disagree
41. Changes introduced at the right time, by the right person, in the right manner, will always be accepted.	❏	❏
42. The timing of a change should be primarily based on the work schedule to support client demands, not the staff schedule.	❏	❏
43. Overcoming resistance to change requires primarily that the boss, administrator, and middle managers know their facts and communicate clearly the logic behind the change.	❏	❏
44. Staff members with negative attitudes toward projected changes should be encouraged to quit.	❏	❏
45. Changes based only on facts and logic will be sabotaged by the staff members whom the change affects.	❏	❏
46. When staff members understand the reasons for a change, they will never resist it.	❏	❏
47. The correct leadership style in dealing with resistance is to be personable, not task oriented.	❏	❏
48. Change should never be implemented by ordering it done.	❏	❏
49. Most resistance within practice organizations is caused by bad relationships and enmity, not simply by inertia.	❏	❏
50. A change that is good for the practice should be pressed home regardless of the political impacts within the team.	❏	❏
51. Internal changes that do not have impact on other areas of the practice can be implemented without clearing them with the boss.	❏	❏
52. Changes that don't cost any money should be implemented without bothering the boss or manager.	❏	❏

	Agree	Disagree
53. Change does not need to be oriented to the core values of the practice group, only to the manager and leader's directions.	❑	❑
54. Change can be obtained either by reducing the costs of the change or increasing the benefits.	❑	❑
55. Most administrators and managers find that it is harder to get change implemented upward with doctors than it is to make changes downward in the staff organization.	❑	❑
56. All change creates unexpected by-products.	❑	❑

READY FOR CHANGE ASSESSMENT
Answers & Discussion

INSTRUCTIONS

The following answers and discussions are meant to enlarge the point made in each of the questions in the assessment. As you read the discussion items, look particularly at the conflicting answers, and ask. "How does this question and discussion apply to our practice?" Then ask, "If we started continuous quality improvement (CQI), how would this question and answer apply to us tomorrow?"

I. Understanding Change

1. **A.** In certain advanced fields like electronics, knowledge is doubling every three to five years, and in veterinary medicine, every two to three years. Job obsolescence is one of the major impacts of the fluid work environment most practices now face. Usually, veterinary practice job descriptions need to change on an evolving basis, based on needs and staff strengths, so that the obsolescence of what the job represented 5 to 10 years ago is not always apparent. Practice managers who perceive the work place as fixed will find themselves in an increasingly uncomfortable role, defending the status quo rather than birthing the future.

2. **DA.** The rate of change when plotted on a graph resembles an increasingly steeper slope. Change is best thought of as a geometric, not an arithmetic, progression in which more and more change must be dealt with in less and less time; the new millennium will seem to take quantum leaps compared to just a decade ago.

3. **DA.** While professional associations, new technology, and practice leaders are major sources of change decisions, client demands and economic pressures are probably more important as source factors.

4. **DA.** Quality of life is perceived by a majority of people to be declining; discretionary dollars are being called upon by more outside sources just for lifestyle distractions. Surveys show that if people had to live at some time other than the present, either in the past or in the future, most would choose to live in the past.

5. **A.** However, the general linearity of change often sees abrupt changes in direction. Studies of history show that various written predictions of what the

future was going to be like never turned out as good or as bad as predicted. Change is often moderated, toned down by societal values, economic forces, and other factors.

6. **A.** New managers are unwilling to confront the boss and need time to gain the trust of the leadership as an independent decision maker. The more experienced practice administrator generally has an agenda that he/she validates during the first year and puts into place and consolidates in the second; in the third year, he/she makes a major run at changing things. This is not to say that managers don't continue to make changes over prolonged assignments, but the peaks are usually lower. Some group administrators play into this phenomenon by deliberately rotating members of their management team(s) to keep the change engine revved up.

7. **DA.** People management, motivation, and dealing with resistance have all been found to require much more work than the technical chores of the change itself. Because this organizational behavior is not well understood by veterinary practice owners, many practice managers have difficulty in change management. The average practice generally falls into the trap of designing the new project in terms of detailed process, but not putting nearly enough work into the human questions surrounding implementation and outcome expectations.

II. The Manager's Role

8. **A.** Given the constant of change, it's unrealistic to think of the job as static or fixed (if you just reacted to the "his" of this question, you are not ready for innovation and creativity—you are focusing on the wrong things). Obviously, this statement calls for some caution to make sure that staff members and the attending doctor understand that case management is strictly the doctor's domain, and the changes you'll be making as a group are in the organizational and operational support of that mission. Also—don't move so abruptly that people take it as a criticism of previous ways of doing things.

9. **A.** While it might be possible to get people to "do what I say, not what I do," it's usually easier to ask people to do what the manager is willing to do on a routine basis, if it is founded in the core values of the practice.

10. **A.** While this may be arguable in specific cases, it appears that management team resistance is the biggest obstacle. Similarly, when a new administrator or new middle managers who are brought on board come to believe in the prac-

tice agenda, a committed leadership group can overcome most other obstacles.

11. **A.** Innovation is one of seven key result areas for any manager. The others are client satisfaction, productivity, quality, economic health, personal growth, and developing a positive organization climate. Practice managers who think that their job is simply to develop forms, write protocol, and run the practice on the straight and narrow as it has always been done, act as a barrier to change, ignoring suggestions from the practice team.

12. **DA.** Resistance is not a sufficient reason by itself to retract a change request. However, if the reasons for resistance are legitimate and substantial, then it may be sensible to retract the change while the team decides on an acceptable alternative to achieve the desired practice expectations.

13. **DA.** This answer assumes that the reason the change isn't working is poor communication or other normal resistance. A change that is simply badly designed should, of course, be tossed out. Whether the old way should be reinstated is doubtful since the need for a new approach had been deemed necessary. Perhaps a third alternative is necessary.

14. **DA.** Studies show that almost all staff members know of at least one thing that can be improved in their "line of sight," the immediate area of their job that they know well. Often ideas are not shared because the management never asks or because the climate, set largely by the doctors and managers, is not conducive to sharing.

III. Encouraging Ideas

15. **A.** Contrary to what some managers believe, staff members will have more respect for the manager who admits a mistake than for one who insists on maintaining the error. Don't let pride get in the way of results.

16. **DA.** One of the bad features of many suggestion box programs is that they by-pass the middle management. Quality circles (or CQI empowerment) avoid this problem, as do suggestion systems that operate informally and continuously within each work area of the practice.

17. **DA.** There's nothing wrong with tangible incentives or cash, but a number of highly successful healthcare systems work well with recognition as the reward. National surveys report that implementation of the idea is the biggest reward in the perception of most employees, regardless of career field.

18. **A.** As a general rule, giving staff members the freedom to take action en-

hances their self-esteem and gives them a sense of control over their job environment. However, it may not be possible on very large or costly projects to do this, so the principle often has to be compromised by the situation.

19. **DA**. Asking people for their ideas and letting them participate in planning the change are powerful ways to gain their receptivity. However, if the supervisor is just going through the motions and is not genuine, this approach will be worthless and may even cause greater resistance later on.

20. **DA**. The answer here is based on a proper quality circle (or project team) implementation. Developing staff teams into semiautonomous work teams is one of the best investments of time a manager can make.

21. **A.** In older, authoritarian management systems, most issues were decided by the managerial elite (e.g., the single doctor, as practice owner); the chain of command arrangement also meant that lower levels were not allowed to make decisions. This concept worked acceptably well as long as there weren't too many decisions. In the current explosion of problems and changes requiring decisions in the new millennium, delegation of operating decisions to the lowest possible levels (accompanied with a lot of training and controlled review of progress to the expected outcome) makes the most sense. Otherwise, management becomes a major bottleneck to progress.

IV. Creating Dissatisfaction

22. **A.** The old concept of organization living was to not rock the boat, that those who did were troublemakers; the concept of the newer era was "If it ain't broke, leave it alone." Neither of these attitudes allows a timely response to changing dynamics in the community or profession. Creative dissatisfaction building is a key managerial skill, since people who are satisfied will not willingly accept change.

23. **A.** In line with the answer above, publicize every possible problem with the current system **without blaming** anyone involved. Address the issues, not the people; look at future needs, not past stumbles. This will at first shock, but then it will help to shift people's mindset toward looking for ways to solve these problems.

24. **A.** This is best in the sense that serving others is a prime motivator for many healthcare workers, and especially for veterinary practice staff. Also, client ratings have often been found to be more valid for practice improvement planning than are reports from finance, quality control, or other sources.

The practice manager's relationship with staff is often protected when an outside group of significant others can be referenced as a source of dissatisfaction. An unhappy client tells a dozen people, and each of those tell five more, while a satisfied client will tell only half a dozen. You do the math, but ensure that the dissatisfied client is contacted by a decision maker within 24 hours and that the issue is resolved.

25. **A.** "If it isn't broken, why fix it?" While we may wish it were otherwise, in most veterinary practices, change does not occur until a bunch of people get unhappy over an issue. In a traditional veterinary practice environment, most staff members are interested in solving a problem so that they will not see it again. Simply improving a currently acceptable situation is seldom seen as a valid reason for the manager to take valuable time away from the healthcare delivery mission.

26. **DA.** Dissatisfaction data drives decisions **only** when the research is politically supported, relevant, and timely. Reports and measures that target individuals are sensed as blaming, and defensiveness replaces change. When positive, issue-based conditions do not accompany data, the data is not considered important information; it's just another academic study.

27. **A.** Unfortunately, many veterinary managers report burnout from repeated efforts to get over the mountain of practice inertia. Running into brick walls tends to be both painful and fatiguing. Wise administrators and leaders will generally push for a limited agenda of priorities across a narrow practice front. This allows task completion and the joy of achievement; behavior rewarded is behavior repeated. Asking people to do too many things at once dissipates energy, and a lot of energy is required for change.

28. **DA.** Successful change managers report that there is invariably a hidden guerrilla army ready to support good change. Often it is underground and quiescent. One of the skills of good change managers is identifying these commandos and enlisting them in their cause. One of the roles of a good consultant is finding the hot buttons of the simmering underground army and empowering them to attack the status quo with a vengeance (directed and paced in conjunction with the transition plan of the practice).

V. Communcation/Participation

29. **DA.** Time allows for adjustments in thinking, attitudes, and behavior. Over 66 percent of the American workforce dislikes change and prefers the status quo; these people need warm-up time to get ready.

30. **DA.** As a general rule, individual communication is better so that the change can be dealt with in terms of each person's reaction to it. Group announcements are sometimes required, but as a general pattern, the blind-side change announcement creates a feeling in staff members that they are only cogs in the great veterinary practice machine. Groups, especially within specific areas of the hospital, are often better when they get to figure out ways to implement and smooth the change process.

31. **A.** While it isn't a hard and fast rule, and while the manager should not defer to the informal group leader, communicating with this person is often an effective way to get the word out. Since the informal group leader is usually respected by the others in the group, the change gains some credibility when it comes from this secondary source.

32. **A.** The motivational force of emotion is far more powerful than that of logic.

33. **DA.** While communication and participation are powerful tools to enlist people's support, there are instances where the proper role of the manager is simply to order immediate change or compliance. Examples might be safety regulations, an immediate external threat, or big financial consequences.

34. **DA.** Try to win over the resistant staff member(s) through persuasion and communication. Do the same with other staff members. Little by little, the unreasonably resistant person will be walled off by the others. Later, if the resistance becomes gross insubordination or undercuts the supervisor, it can be dealt with through disciplinary channels (see the staff development assessment in Appendix E).

35. **DA.** How can people be won over if management and leadership do not stand up for their programs? It's sometimes possible to win them over with a forthright communication effort. Often, however, the real reasons for resistance are rooted in individual attitudes or circumstances that underlie the refusal to consider management's proposal or needs of the practice. Some people are so *me* oriented, that *we* does not exist. If the *power of we* cannot be accepted by specific people on the practice staff, then each person will have to be dealt with using a one-to-one, welcome-to-reality session.

VI. Implementing Change

36. **DA.** The answer here is a judgement call. Giving people time to adjust or time to experiment with the change on a pilot basis is usually better than

immediate implementation. Ninety-day test scenarios often take the threat out of a change scenario, but by the end of the test, the new habits are established and change is no longer an issue. If the situation calls for it, doing the right things, right away, by the right people, may be necessary.

37. **A.** As a general principle, going slowly and allowing people to adjust to unpopular change is the way to proceed in any setting, but it is especially critical in veterinary healthcare delivery where the staff is usually underpaid, under-recognized, and understaffed. If there's no way the staff are going to change their acceptance viewpoint, then it's sometimes better to proceed quickly and decisively.

38. **A.** Not communicating that termination or realignment may be in the works increases suspicion of management and reduces the amount of time that people need to make other job arrangements. De-hiring is a slow process of awareness of outcome expectations and a person's personal acceptance of being in the wrong job, for the wrong reason, at the wrong time. Black Fridays, when the bomb announcement hits fifteen minutes before quitting time, will never be considered fair by those who remain.

39. **A.** If the answer to this question is *Disagree* for your practice, something needs to be done, and soon, to change people's attitudes. When the mission focus and core values become secondary to individual whims, the tail is wagging the dog, and that is a pathologic condition requiring immediate and aggressive treatment.

40. **DA.** One reality in every management situation is the opinions and attitudes of the people who will be affected by the change. Both elements must be considered in arriving at wise decisions. The practice culture is based on the perceptions of people: staff, clients, doctors, and vendors.

41. **DA.** Usually this will be the case, but not always. We are sorry—this is a practice reality.

42. **DA.** Both have to be considered. Judgement will require that sometimes work demands, and other times human needs, will have to be given precedence.

VII.   Overcoming Resistance

43. **DA.** Communicating the rational reasons for change is a business effort that should be done, but it is less important than dealing with the emotional needs of people. Resistance to change is primarily an emotional need, not a

need for more data. Listening, dealing with anxieties, providing managerial support, sharing rewards, and sharing control of the project all may be more important than communication of the facts.

44. **DA.** This answer assumes that other attempts to deal with negative attitudes haven't yet been tried. If other things have been tried (staff development assessment, Appendix E), and what is being dealt with is a sour person, then disciplinary approaches may be necessary, including termination.

45. **A.** Usually the basis of rejection of a change for most people has relatively little to do with facts and logic; fear of the unknown is a great barrier. There is comfort in the status quo; ask the doctors, they will tell you the same thing, "We have **always** done it that way!" There are underlying emotional needs or feelings that usually form the basis for acceptance or denial.

46. **DA.** Emotions still must be handled. Conversely, it is not uncommon for people to accept change that they do not understand at all because of trust in the person recommending it. Clients have this sort of relationship with their doctors, as do many staff members with managers who have earned their respect.

47. **A.** *Personable* is not a specific leadership style, but embraces many of the phases of situational leadership. People and their feelings are always the first concern of a leader—everything else in management is secondary. It's important for managers to be people centered, not task centered, so they can effectively lead the change effort.

48. **DA.** Based on conditions where the group is in a high state of readiness, the best leadership style is to order change. Participation is not always a proper approach, especially in emergency medical and surgical situations. The manager needs to ask, "How directive can I be in this situation? Is this the time to set up another training session?" Situational leadership means that you do what is appropriate to the events at hand.

49. **DA.** There may be a bad set of relationships and other resistance factors, but the major cause of resistance is the comfort of the status quo and the tremendous investment of time and personal effort that people have in the way things are being done. Some traditional managers deliberately build in confusion mechanisms such as organization chart changes, staff rotations, and client evaluations, just to keep things stirred up and give the appearance of change. This process is often a form of paralysis by analysis, which is a true art form in some veterinary practices. If the reorganizations, job redesigns, and client feedback systems are used on a recurring basis, to tailor

the continuous quality improvement (CQI) change process, this makes future change easier because the organization has learned that meaningful change is a constant.

VIII. Influencing Support

50. **A.** The answer here is arguable. Veterinary practice harmony is a day-by-day series of relationship moderations. Occasionally it will cost the manager something to push for change; all decisions have consequences, so that is not a reason to fear pushing for something you believe in. It becomes a matter of personal courage and sensitivity to know when and how much to push and whether the project is worth it. The bottom line is that if managers never pushed except when there were no costs, precious little forward gain would be made for their practice, the staff's development, or their own careers.

51. **A.** This may not be the safe answer based on the relationship you have with your boss, but it is the preferred one. We believe in training to trust; we believe this is a commitment of the leadership in **every** practice. There are too many timorous managers waiting for permission to act, too many bosses creating subordinate cripples; if you cannot trust the staff, the training and leadership are at fault. Continuous quality improvement often means "Just do it!"

52. **A.** As in the above answer, the reason managers are on the payroll is to move things forward. Veterinary practice is generally a series of problems, from clients, staff, doctors, or the community. The assumption in this answer is that the change is sound and not politically stupid.

53. **DA.** Change that violates the practice's core values will ultimately fail. By core values we mean the personal beliefs, bioethics, and integrity of the practice's leadership team. However, change may challenge the norms of the healthcare delivery team in terms of currently accepted definitions of quality, scope of services, quality of care, patient advocacy, and other standards of performance. These norms will be very difficult to change, but may be challenged at times when crises are not being resolved. The core values, on the other hand, must be considered inviolate by every member of the practice. To change these would be to change who the group really is.

54. **A.** To the extent that change resistance is seen as too costly, or as providing little payoff opportunity, most people would prefer to leave things as they

are. One art of change management is to decrease the costs of change and increase the values. At the same time, some managers will seek to increase the costs of not changing, and decrease the benefits of the old system. This is the art and science of management negotiation.

55. **A.** Doctors rise to the top of the practice hierarchy because of professional education; new millennium management includes strength of personality and compassion for others. This professional competency strength in doctors is sometimes a weakness, in that their dedication to certain healthcare delivery goals can blind them to the emerging community needs and practice change options. Part of the problem, too, is that veterinary managers may tend to be overly cautious for the wrong reasons, afraid to tell the emperor that he has no clothes.

56. **A.** No matter how good the planning for change has been, unforeseen results are going to occur. Effective leaders and savvy managers take advantage of the good ones and mediate the bad ones.

WHAT'S NEXT?

What does the number of on-target hits mean in each of the eight sections?
Short Answer—Nothing!

Area of Concern		Number of On-target Hits
I.	Understanding Change	_____
II.	The Manager's Role	_____
III.	Encouraging Ideas	_____
IV.	Creating Dissatisfaction	_____
V.	Communication/Participation	_____
VI.	Implementing Change	_____
VII.	Overcoming Resistance	_____
VIII.	Influencing Support	_____

The above scores are indicators of areas of strengths and of areas needing overt developmental awareness attention. There are no right or wrong answers; assessments are specific to each practice, including where the team is in its own development cycle, where the manager/administrator/leadership sits in the operational parameters, and what the community demands have been. Just be aware of which groups are in the top third (By Jove, I think you've got it!) and which are in the bottom third (We may need help here!). Use available resources to enhance practice awareness of the change process.

APPENDIX A

Nurturing Your Leadership Competencies

Nurture: The act or process of promoting the development of; training.

It is a puzzle faced by every practice leader today: How do you effectively lead a practice team during a time when everything, from structure, to community, to strategies, to values, has dramatically changed? When do you *empower* the employees? When do you *coach* them? When do you *direct* them? When must you *demand*? How do you know which style of leadership is needed?

Leadership strategies shift along with everything else, bringing with them confusing and conflicting changes in terminology and techniques. We are bombarded with exhortations from the total quality management (TQM) movement of industry, the continuous quality improvement (CQI) movement of health care, and the total quality service/total management service (TQS/TMS) copy-cat ideas of lateral organizations. The confusion is compounded by a wide variety of self-appointed management experts. It is no wonder that veterinary practice leaders don't know whether to reengineer their personalities, reinvent the practice organization, or simply become virtuous human beings and try to please everyone in every situation.

Skill Is Not Enough

Inadequate performance in any practice is rarely due to a lack of knowledge or technical skill. Think about deficient managers you have watched in your own practice. More often then not, their failure or inferior performance in a specific position can be traced to the attitudes, motives, style, or personal characteristics upon which they rely to carry out the responsibilities of their jobs. In some cases, the owner has delegated the process, without delegating the authority, responsibility, or accountability to make it better. Worse yet, he/she may have delegated the job without having provided the training. Training to trust prior to delegation will be assumed for the rest of this appendix.

While technical skills and knowledge are indeed important factors in job success, and while they are the visible portion of the manager's capabilities, they represent only the tip of the iceberg. Other factors are less obvious. They lie under the surface, but they are the competencies required for superior results within any team. Competencies can include any trait, behavior, skill, or other personal attribute that permits or nurtures outstanding performance. While some competencies are relatively easy to train and develop, others are deeply embedded traits of an individual that cannot be changed from the outside, regardless of the good intentions of the trainer. They are personal, inner values, learned at an early age or by experience, and can only be tuned by the person him/herself. The best of leaders and trainers can nurture the

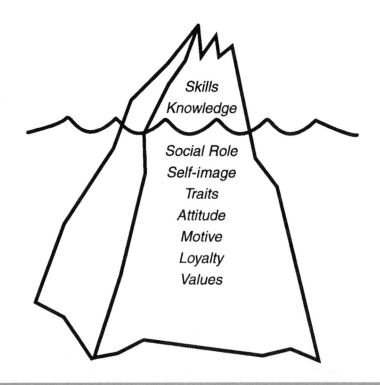

COMPETENCIES ICEBERG

changes, but they can only directly affect the environment. Mothers know it, and scoutmasters practice it: *Behavior rewarded is behavior repeated.* The leader nurtures development (self and others) by rewarding the positive. In his/her quest to modify these inner values of others, the savvy leader sets up discoveries, or capitalizes on an actual event, to engender cognitive awareness in a team member that he/she needs to modify attitudes, behavior, traits, motive, social role, or other leadership competencies.

The visible skills and knowledge of the competencies iceberg are what appear on the resume, and what most veterinarians screen for during candidate interviews. But if the person being added to the team is not also screened for the important underlying competencies, the search will be conducted again in a few months because the person "didn't fit the team" or left because they were uncomfortable with the environment. This same principle applies to leadership and managers already in the practice. The competencies that lie below the surface will be the real determining factors of superior performance, team harmony, and practice success. Nurturing the competencies in self and others is leadership in action and is an operational key to less stress and more harmony.

Competencies for the Future

While it is difficult to predict which leadership competencies will be important in the future of any specific veterinary practice, we can look to the history of successful healthcare organizations and seek models of excellence. In fact, The American College of Healthcare Executives (ACHE) has shown that it is the leadership which makes CQI or TQM programs succeed or fail, not the staff. Uncommon leaders are required to make CQI a successful process. It is the systematic identification of differentiating competencies that makes a competency model more than a simple list of desired attributes and qualities. But a disclaimer is required, even with this approach. In the landmark text of a decade ago, *In Search of Excellence,* 10 industries were held up as models of excellence. But as we entered the 1990s, half of those had fallen on hard times. They had not changed with the society and community they supported. Leadership and excellence are dynamic. Change is the rule, not the exception, and what worked yesterday likely may not work tomorrow. The true leader is rare, but uncommon leadership is what the future requires for continued success in veterinary medicine.

The competencies that lead to superior performance in one practice may or may not lead to superior performance in another. Every veterinary organization has its own culture, its own distinct challenges, and a unique environment. While labels and general descriptions may be the same, *team, leadership, harmony, innovation,* etc., specific behavior indicators will be very different from practice to practice. This is why it is so important to observe and study what people are actually doing to achieve results that are considered superior in our profession.

Given these parameters, it is possible to develop a core set of competencies. These competencies have been selected and modified to reflect the unique challenges inherent in veterinary practice leadership:

Vision

• *The vivid dream.* The uncommon leader is the person who can paint the dream so vividly with words that all around him/her have no doubt where the goal will be.

• *Strategic orientation.* The leader of tomorrow develops and maintains a broad-based, long-term perspective on the mission and the business of veterinary medicine.

• *Conceptual.* The practice leader quickly grasps the connection among diverse ideas, concepts, issues, and events, never blaming others, but rather looking for internal cause-and-effect relationships.

• *Analytical.* The successful practice leader breaks down complex problems, tasks, and projects, into manageable, logically related components, which team members can understand, share ideas about, and develop alternatives for assessment.

Leadership

• *Drive.* Shows an intense personal desire for excellence, wants to lead and motivate others to excel and grow.

• *Change.* Embraces new ideas, expects innovation and creativity, wants people to solve problems at their level, champions CQI in every practice aspect and job position.

• *Harmony.* Models effective leadership in personal behavior, is predictable and dependable, ensures that team actions reflect confidence in staff's ability as well as the individual expertise of team members.

- *Trust.* Shows respect, gives responsibility and accountability for outcomes, recognizes risk takers, gives credit, and takes the blame.

Practice

- *Organizational understanding.* Identifies specific dysfunctional operations, changes jobs to fit the strengths of the individuals, ranks process as secondary to client-centered outcomes.

- *Talent.* Promotes for performance and productivity, not tenure; focuses on staff development and training on a recurring basis, and communicates performance expectations based on developmental growth.

- *Ownership.* Involvement and accountability are reflected in the placement of decision making at the lowest staff level possible. Initiative, self-direction, and unilateral decisions based on what is right for the situation are encouraged.

- *Belonging.* Sense of being needed and trusted is felt at all levels, competency is the daily goal, participation is recognized and specifically appreciated on a daily basis.

Results

- *Achievement.* Continually strives to maximize limited resources to achieve higher quality results for client and patient.

- *Bias for action.* Balances need for consensus and involvement with the need for decisiveness and action. Believes *luck* means being ready to grab an opportunity as it passes by.

- *Accountability.* Provides clear and specific expectations for outcomes, holds self and staff accountable to agreed-upon goals and objectives. Accepts personal accountability for poor levels of training expertise within the team.

- *Recognition.* Seeks to commend unique and creative actions, tailors the reward to the individual, makes practice improvement fun, and ensures at least 60 percent of the staff can be winners.

Self-action

- *Self-confidence.* Projects strong belief in own ideas and abilities without being arrogant.

- *Responsibility.* Internally accepts accountability for everything that affects the practice; does not blame others inside or outside the practice; is accountable for solutions, not excuses.

- *Commitment.* Aligns personal priorities and behavior with the mission, balances home life and practice, yields personal bias to the good of the practice and/or client.

- *Insight.* Exhibits desire and openness to learn from others and from experience. Continually works toward growth and development of self and interteam relationships.

Levels of Team Leadership

While the qualities cited above provide a general framework for relevant leadership competencies, they do not include the level of behavioral detail required for accurate measurement and development guidance that differs significantly from practice to practice. The diagram of the levels of team leadership shown below provides a yardstick for measuring the development of the uncommon leader needed in veterinary practice today.

The Levels 1 to 12 in the diagram reflect an increasing proficiency in team leadership. When someone classifies his/her comfort zone at level 8 or level 9, the levels between the current rating and level 12 reflect competencies and traits that need to be pursued, nurtured, and practiced. The comfort zone must be stretched with recurring applications of new skills and competencies until they become the new standard.

Some practice leaders do not have an accurate mirror to look into on a regular basis. They need to develop a survey using the competency models, the levels scale, and most often, an outside consultant skilled in leadership assessment. The survey is for staff and associates to use to target the leadership style(s) usually seen in the practice day. This evaluation tool is a good team builder if the boss is willing to listen. Good communication means the ability to listen, to hear what is really being said, and to understand that no one in the practice really wants to hurt its success since each person's career relies on the practice becoming better.

LEVELS OF LEADERSHIP

12   **LEADS**—has genuine charisma.

11   Positions self as leader, ensures everyone buys into mission, oversees group tasks.

10   Acts to protect group, gathers right people, resources, and information for the team.

9   Uses complex strategies to promote teamwork and cooperation in hiring and discipline decisions, team assignments—cross-training required.

8   Uses power and authority in fair and equitable manner.

7   Publicly gives credit to others. Encourages and empowers others. Promotes friendly climate, good morale, and cooperation.

6   **FACILITATES**—Values others' input and expertise, ensures everyone contributes, encourages initiative.

5   Expresses positive expectations of others, speaks of subordinates in positive manner, respects others and appeals to their reason.

4   Keeps people informed and up to date, communicates clear, concise expectations.

3   **MANAGES**—Manages meetings and projects. States agendas and objectives, controls time, and makes assignments. Trains to task.

2   Cooperates, participates willingly.

1   **PARTICIPATES**—Participates reluctantly, is burnout and a footdragger.

0   Neutral-passive, does not participate—abdicates.

−1   Disruptive, uncooperative, causes conflict and disharmony.

Unlocking Potential

The key to leadership growth and development is accurate and focused feedback. As an instructor of over a dozen leadership courses, over half of which were in a high adventure, outdoor format, I have come to see very clearly that the quality of performance feedback is inversely related to one's organizational level. The barriers to feedback are broken down when an outside facilitator enters the group. The higher you are, the less truth people are willing to share about your behavior and attitudes. In fact, veterinary practice owners, association executive directors, and even practice administrators are very vulnerable to misleading and inaccurate input regarding personal style, cognitive ability, leadership effectiveness, and organizational savvy.

The competencies described here can provide a head start to developing a plan and a process that will ensure meaningful and relevant goals. If the staff is nurtured and rewarded for participating in the new developmental process, feedback quality will improve, and the leader will become better. As the leadership improves, so does the delegation and sharing of accountability by the team. As the team accepts accountability, responsibility, and ownership for their corners of the practice, continuous quality improvement and problem prevention will become the standard. Progress will replace status quo, change will replace inertia, and net growth will replace gross growth without net. The times will be easier, the team will be happier, and stress will come into perspective.

Ten Areas of Group Administrator Expertise

When in doubt, ask the staff—they know what is needed!
—Dr. T.E. Catanzaro

As the only board-certified veterinarian in the American College of Healthcare Executives, my perspective may be slanted. I believe there is a difference between hospital management, practice management, business management, and being a healthcare administrator. Managers deal with programs and process; administrators deal with outcomes, getting things done through other people, and the use of leadership skills.

The 10 Areas of Concern

As a consultant, and as a healthcare administrator, I find the old school demands a job description. I consider a *job description* simply to be a statement of the minimum standards of training required during the introductory period of employment. A better set of parameters lies within the *job standards*, which are the outcome expectations created by those who do the hiring. Since each practice has different expectations, the standards are not cookie-cutter clean, but the areas of interest are. I see 10 major areas of professional development that are required for any veterinary hospital administrator. These are

- Governance
- Organization arrangements
- Bioethics and practice values
- Planning
- Marketing
- Human resources

- Financial assessment

- Facility planning

- Professional education

- Quality improvement

John Griffith's reference text *The Well-Managed Community Hospital* (Third edition, Chicago: Health Administration Press, 1996) provides a complete integrated overview of the environment and activities of a well-managed facility. There is not a similar comprehensive reference in veterinary medicine, although there are many references (and quick-fix gimmicks) that are "a mile wide and an inch deep." For the purposes of any specific veterinary medical practice, key taskings can be asked for in each of the 10 areas, and the practice-specific answers should provide the job description/job standards required for effective middle management leadership and facility operations.

Organization

- Interpret the practice's role with respect to health service values.

- Define the organization's mission and practice philosophy.

- Ensure effective admission and disposition of patients and their stewards.

- Develop the criteria for evaluation of management efforts.

- Evaluate the internal policies and procedures relative to the practice goals and objectives.

- Report organizational performance to the owners.

- Develop criteria to evaluate owner performance toward practice and staff.

- Assess the impact of change on the motivation of the work groups in the practice.

- Set standards of action required to achieve goals.

Governance

- Be able to explain in detail the difference between policy and implementation, and accept that the role of the board or ownership is to set the standards.

- Explain the implementation requirements for the practice's annual budget and long-term (three- to five-year) plan.

- Develop an organizational structure, delineating accountabilities and authority, which meets the practice's mission.

- Formulate and promulgate policies and procedures which concern professional responsibilities of the practice.

- Help define and establish a set of core values that translates practice theory into action at the staff operational level.

- Provide orientation and direction for professional members of staff.

Organization Arrangements

- Identify the presence and function of other veterinary providers in the area.

- Develop informal cooperative relationships with other veterinary providers, agencies, and specialists.

- Negotiate formal affiliations (contracts).

- Ensure a continuity of care and a medical record accountability system are established and maintained.

- Develop informal linkages with educational institutions.

- Establish appropriate linkages with various advocacy groups.

- Assess the technology impact and potentials for the practice.

- Ensure organizational arrangements for legal counsel.

- Ensure organizational arrangements for internal control audits.

- Identify and evaluate state-of-the-art computer technology.

- Establish information system (computer) support program.

- Ensure integrated systems and data gathering occur within the practice.

Bioethics and Practice Values

- Assess current demographic impact of community on practice.

- Review clinical ethical issues and initiate appropriate action.

- Establish and ensure a routine peer review of veterinary healthcare delivery is conducted and documented, in practice and by medical record audit.

- Identify and respond to conflict-of-interest situations.

- Keep informed of criteria and standards of veterinary healthcare delivery.

- Review business ethical issues and initiate appropriate action.

- Understand and implement grief and stress counseling for clients and staff.

- Develop and promote policies, procedures, and practices that balance the needs of management, providers, clients, and patients.

- Interpret medical/professional staff conduct on behalf of the practice.

Planning

- Implement the organization's mission statement.

- Establish an internal and external communications plan.

- Plan for timely client access, effective examination room utilization, efficient surgical suite obligation, and staff-doctor-client-patient interactions.

- Analyze community needs and demands for veterinary services.

- Ensure a supply and replacement program is developed with multiple vendors to maintain an appropriate cost of goods sold.

- Assess the needs and initiate the training programs required to enhance the capabilities of the staff and practice.

- Ensure consistency between long-range and short-range goals.

- Assess the economic resources available for daily operations.

- Eliminate or modify unproductive programs based on sociological, economic, and political considerations.

- Involve all team members in planning to achieve goals and objectives.

- Evaluate the implications of eliminating a program on the practice's continued success and survival.

- Identify measures by which practice performance can be measured.

- Assess human resource strengths and availability for the practice.

Marketing

- Assess the use of public relations, marketing, and advertising to meet practice goals and objectives.

- Differentiate between internal promotions and external marketing.

- Establish the appropriate internal and external promotion plans to meet the wants and needs of the practice, providers, and clients.

- Assess the cost benefit of specific programs in relation to client benefit and staff benefit assessments.

- Select multiple methods and implement programs to measure client satisfaction with the practice.

- Identify and initiate target marketing efforts and promotions to established and/or potential clients.

- Determine methods to increase client and patient return rates and track successful implementation.

Human Resources

- Establish a human resource philosophy to motivate team members.

- Promote human resource philosophy through practice structure and policies.

- Evaluate alternative compensation and benefit programs.

- Develop criteria for an effective staff benefits and responsibilities manual.

- Identify and assign outcome areas of accountability, ensuring authority and responsibility are delegated to achieve success.

- Evaluate performance and productivity at all levels.

- Assess manpower needs, including skills assessment and shift demands.

- Ensure consistency between practice policies and existing laws.

- Plan for effective practice scheduling of staff members.

- Promote teamwork and motivation within the staff members.

- Arbitrate matters of dispute between staff members to achieve proper operational effectiveness.

- Develop an outplacement program for terminated staff members.

Financial Assessment

- Establish a capital equipment demand list and provide it to the ownership.

- Implement the AAHA chart of accounts and financial accounting system.

- Plan program-based budgets to reflect the income to expense balance required for quality patient care, liquidity, and client bonding.

- Develop workload forecasts, cash flow projections, and program-based needs for practice success in sequential periods of operation.

- Respond to external forces that diminish the practice's assets.

- Develop a system to ensure confidentiality of business records are maintained.

- Utilize trend analyses and fiscal factors to assess profitability of programs, people, and the practice.

- Develop business plans to enhance new program planning and implementation.

- Evaluate the operating budget relative to practice goals and actual achievements.

- Initiate variance analyses as needed to ensure negative trends can be addressed and reversed in a timely manner.

- Develop an integrated system to control accounts receivable.

- Utilize cost-finding methods to assist in decision making.

- Recommend rate structures and fee schedules which marry the philosophy of ownership with the wants and needs of clients and staff.

Facility Planning

- Develop a master site plan based on long-range practice goals.

- Plan for proper maintenance of the physical facility and equipment.

- Determine alternative flow patterns which enhance productivity, performance, and client friendliness.

- Develop the pro formas and program the purchase of capital expense and facility improvements required to increase effectiveness.

- Ensure proper procedures for storage and movement of drugs, supplies, and equipment.

- Implement the required procedures and policies for making minor alterations and improvements.

Professional Education

- Establish an appropriate, monthly, in-service continuing education program for staff and providers.

- Review the professional trends and schedule programs enhancing continuation education experiences outside the facility.

- Ensure appropriate literature is available and reviewed in a timely manner.

- Assess the impact of technology on existing programs and policies; ensure changes are initiated to provide liability protection and enhanced care.

- Encourage staff to participate in continuing education and promote literature review discussions to evaluate comprehension and implementation.

- Motivate professionals and paraprofessionals by appealing to their sense of pride and professionalism.

Quality Assessment/Improvement

- Review quality assessment methodologies and develop a team methodology to initiate improvements.

- Implement, evaluate, and monitor the risk management program (OSHA, safety, radiation protection, zoonotic disease, etc.).

- Ensure each client's and each staff member's dignity and safety.

- Analyze various reports relating to quality improvement to ensure desired outcomes are being achieved (pursued).

- Ensure adequacy, confidentiality, and availability of all patient/client care documentation.

- Select methods to measure the quality of services being provided.

- Be aware of all regulatory requirements (DEA, FDA, EPA, OSHA, etc.) and ensure appropriate programs are established to protect staff and practice.

- Develop a program for managers and providers to independently improve the quality of services and care being offered and delivered.

- Establish an on-going patient advocacy and client relations feedback program.

- Discuss identified problems in patient care, facility safety, or other quality standards/regulations with medical/professional staff and reach commitments for outcome changes.

- Implement a quality improvement process within the practice.

- Be prepared to participate with respective staff members in taking corrective actions required for quality improvements.

- Provide reports to the governing body on results of quality improvements.

The Rest of the Story

With all of the above rhetoric, a quality administrator is still not defined. We can, however, use all the phrases that have made consulting famous:

- No one on the staff will care how much the administrator knows until they know how much the administrator cares.

- Managers will take credit and give blame while leaders give credit and take the blame.

- The respect required to be effective is born in caring.

- The "L" in quality stands for leadership.

- Leaders only can establish the environment for motivation; the good team members find the key within themselves.

They all say the same thing, but in different ways; leadership is the common key to veterinary healthcare administration. Innovation and creativity is most often stifled by managers and enhanced by leaders. So the final elements of any job description/job standard needs to end with two calls to action:

- Meet the challenge—solve the problem!

- Challenge the system—make the improvement!

The Annual Business of Business

The ultimate inspiration is the deadline.
—Nolan Bushnell

Yearly Reviews

The end of the calendar year is a celebration time, but it also marks the end of the fiscal year for many veterinary practices. With IRS ruling 92-65 (see *JAVMA*, 201(6), September 15, 1992; *JAVMA*, 206(3), February 1, 1995), it appears accrual accounting is here for tax reporting purposes. Many practices have also started to review their corporate structure each year (this is the law in most states). The last quarter of every year is the time to review certain business items, for management concerns as well as corporate charter requirements. The owners of a veterinary practice should hold a meeting **every** year and review 14 basic business areas (listed below).

Most corporations (and most LLCs) are required to hold an annual meeting of stockholders. The date and time of the meeting are generally set forth in the by-laws of the corporation, and the announcement of the meeting can be waived in writing by the attendees. Even when there is no corporate structure, the annual meeting is needed to review the preceding year's operations and to develop a program-based budget and operations plan for the year to come. For that matter, due to the dynamic nature of a program-based budget (client centered, as in the phrase, "the front door must swing"), the system requires at least quarterly trend reviews at the leadership level of the practice.

Areas for Review

The list provided below represents items that need to be considered by the key decision makers and managers of any veterinary practice, large animal or small, specialist or generalist, corporate or privately held. While it is not an exhaustive list, it outlines matters that are relevant to the business of veterinary practice. In many cases, minutes of these discussions are particularly important in cases of a lawsuit or an Internal Revenue Service examination.

- Financial assessment of balance sheets and income statements of the preceding year. Conduct a fiscal analysis of the practice operations.

- Election of directors/officers, if corporate.

- Prior year compensation formulas.

- Next year staffing needs and compensation formulas.

- Deferred compensation plans (and other retirement packages).

- Loan status.

- Banking needs and support assessment.

- Extraordinary corporate actions (legal structure demands, e.g., IRS 92-65).

- Fringe benefits (health insurance, medical reimbursement plans, CE).

- Document review (tax returns, investment reports, state licensure, etc.).

- Compliance review (trade name, COBRA, I-9s, OSHA, ADA, DEA, FDA, employment laws, discrimination policies, and other record-keeping needs).

- Proper use of practice name and logo (corporate name and mark).

- Short-term planning (program-based budgeting, income center to cost center, marketing needs, facility space reallocation, communication plan, transition plan for year, etc.).

- Long-term planning (three-year business plan, renovations, expansions, etc.).

The importance of reviewing and making decisions in the above areas, as well as recording them, cannot be emphasized too much. The joint discussions get the team on the right track and integrate the business of operating a veterinary practice with the quality of healthcare delivery. They do go together!

A corporation can lose its corporate status and thus its limited liability as a result of neglecting these matters. On audit, an IRS agent
will ask to inspect the corporate minutes, and if matters such as the
proper recording of a loan to an owner/officer are not in order, the IRS
could deem the loan a taxable cash dividend. Another common example of the importance of maintaining corporate minutes is the proper
recording of salary increases or bonuses to key employees, so that the
IRS doesn't regard this as a dividend, and therefore tax it twice.

Mid-year Tax Reviews

To get ready for the end-of-year planning process, mid-year reviews
are beneficial, especially for tax purposes. This is more than the capital expense budget (mid-year equipment procurement actions are often
tax benefits looking to happen as well as income center supports) and
can be done concurrently with the quarterly review of the program-
based budget by the practice leadership. The mid-year tax position review must look forward and center on greater tax liability forecasting
(e.g., depreciation and amortization schedules, investment credits, retirement funds, corporate restructuring, etc.). The following concepts
need to be discussed with your accountant, preferably at mid-year, so
there is maneuvering space:

Individual

- Review of withholding and estimated tax payments (e.g., must be at
  least 90 percent of 1994 tax bill).

- Make retirement plan contributions [e.g., IRA, SEP, 401(k), Keogh,
  etc., provide accumulated tax free earnings until withdrawal].

- Maximize deductions (e.g., medical over 7.5 percent of adjusted
  gross, miscellaneous over 2 percent of adjusted gross).

- Check out tax-favored investments (depends most on overall financial picture).

- Donate to charity (e.g., unneeded treasures to charity for fair market value (FMV) deduction).

- Restructure your debt (e.g., home-equity loan is one of the last re-
  maining tax write-offs, unlike credit cards, car loans, and other con-
  sumer debts).

Practice

- Plan equipment purchases (e.g., federal-credit equipment deduction versus depreciation).

- Shift income and deductions (e.g., defer income or accelerate tax deductible expenses—but if done every year, as for large end-of-year drug purchases, it only affects the first year).

- Estimate your tax bill accurately (especially important for sole proprietors, partners, and Sub-S corporations—be aware of any defined breakpoint).

- Review business meals and entertainment (e.g., audit hot spot since, effective December 31, 1993, deduction became only 50 percent).

- Write off bad debts promptly (e.g., deductions can **only** be taken in the year when a debt officially becomes worthless).

- Don't overlook tax credits (e.g., targeted job credits).

Summary

A veterinary practice can lose its focus, on the business of practice as well as on the healthcare delivery quality and client-centered service. To deal with this loss of focus, there is an integrated system for doing program-based budgeting. Although the accountant should be skilled at the above tax issues and be able to convert cash-based daily operations to accrual for tax purposes, most accountants don't understand the veterinary practice programs which produce the income. Therefore, program-based activities require leadership from a veterinary professional.

During these recessionary times, there are many practice owners who have started to focus so tightly on the bottom line that they have lost sight of client and patient needs. There are also many associate veterinarians and other staff members (usually very underpaid) who have lost sight of the business and in their caring have given away the practice net. This annual mid-year and year-end exercise allows both business and need perspectives to be addressed and requires a consensus on the integration of these perspectives for the coming year. Wouldn't that be nice in your practice?

Understanding Behavioral Patterns

Behavior is a mirror in which everyone displays his image.
—Johann Goethe

Psychologists believe that the reactive behavior pattern you feel most comfortable with was established by the time you were 12. This bit of knowledge should not make a hospital director feel too happy, to be surrounded by 12-year-olds during times of stress. On the other hand, it may be a reason to put fun back into practice!

Developed Behavior Patterns

As we have grown to the adults we are today, we have attempted to be what we thought we should have become. This is another challenge, since it is often based on the perceptions and feedback from others, and may conflict with personal preferences. The results of all these outside influences are "developed behavior patterns"—distinct ways of thinking, feeling, and acting. The central core of our patterns tends to remain stable because it reflects our individual identities. However, the demands of the veterinary practice environment often require different responses that evoke into a work behavioral style.

The traditional Myers-Briggs system is a personality profile and almost impossible for a veterinary practice leader to self-administer. The more friendly Personal Profile System (D-I-S-C) can be evaluated and profiled by a caring practice leader, and aids in understanding work behavior patterns, which are a mix and match of four basic groups:

- *Dominance.* Emphasis is on shaping the environment by overcoming opposition to accomplish results.

- *Influence.* Emphasis is on shaping the environment by bringing others into alliance to accomplish results.

- *Steadiness*. Emphasis is on cooperating with others on the team to carry out the task.

- *Conscientious*. Emphasis is on working with existing circumstances to promote quality in products or service.

Interestingly, as described above, each personality pattern has some behavior characteristics that could help a practice. So why doesn't everyone get along? Because each person is a mixture of the patterns, and each has strengths, fears, limitations, and different motivators. The astute manager will learn these factors and use them to the practice's advantage. The following description of work behavior tendencies briefly expands on these D-I-S-C factors for each behavior tendency. It is a simplified chart showing how the primary behavior pattern of any staff member should be used to change the management approach to that individual. While it is not the intent to change the practice owner's personality profile, an awareness of others' behavior preferences makes the communication effort a lot easier. It usually gets results quicker, also.

Work Behavior Tendencies

High 'D' Work Behavior Tendencies

- Strengths   Decisiveness, high energy, competitiveness
                   High sense of personal worth, natural leader
                   Task(end result)-oriented, problem-solving

- Motivations   Directness, power

- Fear   Being taken advantage of

- Limitations   Impatience, overruns people, too blunt

- Weaknesses   May try to do it all themselves
                   May not let good people do the job
                   May neglect small details, opinions of other

- Frequency   Makes up about 17 percent of the American
                   workforce

High 'I' Work Behavior Tendencies

- Strengths   Persuasive, positive, enthusiastic, cooperating, poised
                Optimistic, people-oriented relaters, social-oriented, trusting

- Motivations   Social recognition, acceptance

- Fear   Social rejection

- Limitations   Disorganization, time problems, easy mark

- Weaknesses   Trusts others rather than checking details
                Talks too much, oversells ideas, tells secrets
                Too many meetings, poor time management
                Delays the difficult or unpleasant

- Frequency   Makes up about 17 percent of the American workforce

High 'S' Work Behavior Tendencies

- Strengths   Dependable, loyal, productive, predictable, pragmatic, calm
                Technical competence, team player, friendly, patient
                Concrete systematic approach, sticking to it

- Motivations   Traditional practices, loyalty

- Fears   Loss of stability, break of tradition

- Limitations   Slow to change, adheres to code of "order and tranquility"

- Weaknesses   Hard to share a process, do busy work to feel needed
                Excessively security conscious, withholds information
                Overly involved to point of interference
                May try to let time solve long-range problems

- Frequency   Makes up about 50 percent of the American workforce

High 'C' Work Behavior Tendencies

- Strengths   Accurate, diplomatic, follows directions
                     Handles details, systematic, quality control

- Motivations   "Correct" or "proper" way, precision work

- Fears   Criticism of their work, losing control

- Limitations   Procrastination, overly critical

- Weaknesses   May not trust intuitive abilities
                     Lack of self-confidence, folds under attack
                     Intolerant of ambiguity or uncertainty

- Frequency   Makes up about 17 percent of the American
                     workforce

QUICK D-I-S-C PRIMER

D & I are change agents.   S & C are status-quo supporters.

D & C are task-oriented.   I & S are people-oriented.

The American workforce is 50   D, I, and C are 17 percent each.
percent High S.

S & C make up 66 percent of
the American workforce, so
expect slow change.

A Personal Profile System

There are multiple instruments on the market to help the hospital director become aware of his/herself and others within the practice environment. The hospital director is the central focus for the practice style and philosophy of practice and can greatly influence the practice environment to make it conducive to success. The Personal Profile System (D-I-S-C), published by Carlson Learning Centers and Performax Systems International, has become the instrument used most often by the practice consultants at Catanzaro & Associates, Inc., as well as by the

Veterinary Hospital Managers Association (VHMA), the **only** group that tests then certifies practice managers (Certified Veterinary Practice Manager—CVPM) from within a peer-review environment.

We feel the D-I-S-C is easy to administer, replicable by the practice management, and adequately detailed to allow the user to learn about the differences of others and about the environment they require for maximum productivity and harmony in the practice organization. The behavior pattern descriptions in the next section illustrate some strategies for blending that may be useful.

Strategies for Blending

Dominance

- *Remember a high 'D' may want:* authority, challenges, prestige, freedom, varied activities, difficult assignments, status, logical approaches, opportunity for advancement, power.

- *Manager's secret tools:* Provide direct answers, be brief and to the point, ask *what* questions (not *how*), stick to business. Outline possibilities for the person to get results, solve problems, be in charge. Stress logic of ideas or approaches. When in argument, agree with facts and idea, not the person. If time lines or sanctions exist, get them into the open but relate them to end results or goals (never the process).

Influence

- *Remember a high 'I' may want:* social recognition, popularity, people to talk to, freedom of speech, freedom from control and detail, favorable working conditions, recognition of abilities, to help others, a chance to motivate people.

- *Manager's secret tools:* Provide favorable friendly environment with a chance for the person to verbalize about ideas, people, and his/her intuition. Use testimonials from experts. Provide ideas for transferring talk to action, testimonials of experts on ideas. Provide details in writing but don't dwell on them. Provide time for stimulating and fun activities. Provide democratic relationship, incentives for asking to take on tasks.

Steadiness

- *Remember a high 'S' may want:* status quo, security of situation, time to adjust, appreciation, identification with the group, a work pattern, limited territory, areas of specialization, tradition.

- *Manager's secret tools:* Provide a sincere, personal, and agreeable environment, sincere interest in him/her as a person. Ask *how* questions to get his/her opinions. Present ideas or departures from the status quo in a nonthreatening manner; give the person a chance to adjust. Clearly define roles and goals and his/her place in the plan. Provide personal assurance of support. Emphasize how his/her actions will minimize personal risk. Be patient in drawing out the person's goals and objectives.

Conscientiousness

- *Remember a high 'C' may want:* security, no sudden changes, personal autonomy, attention to his/her objectives, little responsibility, exact job descriptions, status quo, controlled work environment, reassurance, to be part of a group, precision work, finish job.

- *Manager's secret tools:* Take time to prepare your case in advance, provide factual pros and cons of an idea, support ideas with accurate data. Provide reassurance that surprises will not occur. Provide an exact job description with a precise explanation of how it fits, and a step-by-step approach to goals. If agreeing, be specific; if disagreeing, disagree with facts, not the person. Be prepared to provide many explanations in a patient, persistent manner.

Compatibility

The mixing of staff members with different personality types can be either a major benefit to the practice or a disaster. Appendix D.4 is a chart that shows which behavior patterns are compatible and which are not. This chart alone makes the use of a personal profile system a critical element to practice team building.

The Personal Profile System (D-I-S-C) is not a test. You cannot fail. There is no best pattern. Research has shown that the most effective people know themselves, know the demands of the situation, and adapt strategies to meet those needs. The D-I-S-C system assists in key areas of practice operations:

- Identifying personal work behavior styles.

- Creating a motivational environment conducive to success.

- Increasing your appreciation of different work styles.

- Identifying and minimizing potential conflicts with others.

- Developing improved staff interaction and harmony.

Utilization

The D-I-S-C Personal Profile System can be self-administered as well as self-developed, or it can be facilitated by an outside consultant if the consultant is aware of the unique nature of a veterinary practice team. The D-I-S-C system is a communication tool that opens the door to greater understanding of self and others in order to build and maintain a sense of personal worth and self-esteem in the practice. It makes discussing personalities an acceptable action, as in, "Hey boss, your 'C' is showing" or "Please get your 'D' out of here and come back when your 'I' wants to talk." When used effectively, the D-I-S-C system has developed the practice's most precious resource—people—and has significantly improved the upward success spiral of the staff and the practice.

This type of behavior pattern assessment program has been tested and proven effective in the following areas: training and development, coaching and counseling, hiring and placement, performance and production appraisals, career path planning, team building, and even conflict resolution. It should be a tool in the bag of tricks of any hospital director who wishes to develop a winning team and a dynamic veterinary medical practice.

Appendix D.1

The High/Low Combinations of Behavioral Tendencies

In evaluating the fit between the person and the role (ability to do task/job), behavioral tendencies must be understood before expectations can be clearly defined and jointly agreed upon.

Creativity   High D/Low I
Tends to be logical, critical, and incisive in approach to attaining goals. Would be most challenged by problems requiring original or analytical efforts. May become blunt and critical with people. A good new practice builder.

Drive   High D/Low S
Responds quickly to a challenge by mobility and flexibility in approach. Tends to be a versatile self-starter who responds rapidly to competition, even in new situations. A great Emergency Clinic person.

Individuality   High D/Low C
Moves forward directly, even in the face of opposition. A forceful individual who will take a stand and openly contest for their position. Willing to take chances, may even overstep prerogatives. The best solo practitioner model.

Goodwill   High I/Low D
Tends to behave in a poised, cordial manner displaying social assertiveness in situations perceived to be favorable and unthreatening. Tends to exude warmth and strives to establish rapport in first contacts with people. A great admissions receptionist.

Contact   High I/Low S
Tends to seek out people through enthusiasm and spark. An outgoing person who tends to display confidence, often attempting to win people through persuasiveness or emotional appeal. A great person for telephone recalls or telemarketing efforts.

Self-confidence   High I/Low C
Displays self-confidence in endeavors with others, striving to win others over. Likely to feel that, despite what situations may arise, he/she will be able to attain success. A great patient advocate. A good discharge receptionist. The new AAHA practice consultant profile.

Patience   **High S/Low D**

Tends to be a steady, consistent individual who prefers to deal with one assignment at a time. Will usually direct actions into areas requiring specialization. Tends to react steadily under pressure; strives to stabilize environment and is likely to be unfavorable toward sudden or large-scale changes. The trustworthy surgeon.

Reflection (Concentration)   **High S/Low I**

Tends to be patient and controlled. Moves with moderation and deliberateness in undertakings. Will usually project a relatively unruffled appearance. Generally approaches situations with concentration to details involved. The great kennel master or animal caretaker.

Persistence   **High S/Low C**

Tends to be a persistent, preserving individual who is not easily swayed once his/her mind is made up. Will set his/her own pace and stick with it. Can be rigid when force is applied to make moves. A type of person you want to put in accounts receivable.

Adaptability   **High C/Low D**

Tends to act in a careful, measured manner which is responsive to the modifications or compromises required to achieve goals. May appear arbitrary and unbending in following a set rule or formula. Prefers an atmosphere free from personal antagonism and desires activity-focused harmony. A good treatment room staff member.

Perfectionism   **High C/Low I**

Tends to be a stickler for quality assurance systems and processes. Makes decisions based on proven precedent and known facts. Tries meticulously to meet standards established either by self or others. An AAHA inspector of yesteryear. A good laboratory technician.

Sensitivity   **High C/Low S**

Tends to be concerned with avoiding risks and troubles. Tends to look for hidden meanings. Tension may be evident, particularly when under stress for results. Generally, uneasiness is evident until absolute confirmation of the correctness of his/her action or decision has been made. A good maintenance person.

Ambivalence   **C and D Match**

When both C and D are **high**, striving for accomplishment and quality are equal. This type is seen as decisively perfection seeking; will not accept **an** answer to a problem, but rather requires **the** best answer. Person also often indicates a difficulty in making decisions, especially under stress. External signs of this situation are manifested by increased tension and vacillation.

When both C and D are **low**, resistance to demands for personal initiative increases. Prefers to operate independently, but is not inclined to fight for independence. May be unwilling to go along with suggestions from others, even though he/she may not have an alternative plan to propose.

Either of these matching profiles could become destructive to a team building effort if not managed in a very astute manner.

Appendix D.2

Behavioral Demands of Specific Positions

Certain positions within a veterinary practice define themselves, based on demands and/or practice philosophy. We need to fit the right people into the right roles if we want them to succeed *and* enjoy their work. The position descriptions provided below are a starting point for using the D-I-S-C profile to increase job role rewards for team members:

High D positions demand
- getting results
- accepting challenges
- making decisions
- reducing costs
- solving problems

Low D positions demand
- protected environment
- direction
- exercising caution
- deliberating before deciding
- weighing pros and cons

High I positions demand
- contacting people
- motivating others
- helping people
- exhibiting poise
- generating enthusiasm
- speaking well

Low I positions demand
- concentration
- sincerity
- reflection
- working alone
- preference for "things"
- thinking logically

High S positions demand
- performing to standards
- exhibiting patience
- developing special skills
- concentration
- staying in one place
- loyalty

Low S positions demand
- keeping many projects going
- seeking variety
- dissatisfaction with status quo
- reacting quickly to change
- applying pressure
- being flexible

High C positions demand
- following directions
- concentration on details
- being diplomatic
- adhering to procedures
- avoiding trouble
- controlling quality

Low C positions demand
- assuming authority
- acting independently
- facing up to problems
- stating unpopular positions
- delegating
- acting without precedent

Appendix D.3

Expectations of Manager Profile Types

To simplify the guessing process, this appendix tries to outline the usual managerial expectations within each personality type. It is important to understand the operational expectations when trying to understand the individual **or** when the staff member is trying to please the leader/manager.

The High D **manager wants** competence and results.

Low D	no quotas.
High I	recognition and freedom.
Low I	no personal competition.
High S	friendship and harmony.
Low S	immediate results.
High C	predictable and organized support.
Low C	freedom from controls.

When delegating

the High D **manager**	can't delegate (can't wait or trust others).
High I	overdelegates (too optimistic, poor facts).
High S	doesn't delegate (keeps self secure and needed).
High C	reluctantly delegates (then oversupervises).

When communicating

the High D **manager**	is brief and one way.
High I	is lengthy and tells too much.
High S	is stingy and only tells what must be said.
High C	is long-winded and full of details, and communicates in writing.

For time control

the High D **manager**	spends time fighting fires and not planning.
High I	wastes time (with people) and overcommits.
High S	works on a schedule and at a definite pace.
High C	bogs down in detail.

When making decisions

the High D **manager**	is impulsive, without much discussion.
High I	has lots of discussion, avoids tough decisions.
High S	is rigid, stubborn, focused on technical aspects.
High C	wants only low-risk decisions.

When directing people

the High D **manager**	drives rather than leads.
High I	depends on personality, likes one on one.
High S	is too lenient, prefers to ask (not tell).
High C	is very strict but depends on orders from above.

With limitation under pressure

the High D **manager**	reacts too quickly, creates fear without knowing it.
High I	has poor follow-through, loses time control.
High S	resists change, becomes stubborn, procrastinates.
High C	worries, hesitates, confuses, using half-truths.

The aggressive techniques used by

the High D **manager**	are overt: "the ulcer carrier."
High I	are verbal: "the great persuader."
High S	are passive: "a sit-in demonstrator."
High C	are defensive: "the rules say so."

The job satisfaction for

the High D **manager wants**	challenges.
Low D	peace.
High I	recognition.
Low I	things, not people.
High S	security.
Low S	results.
High C	rules.
Low C	personal ways and methods.

Tough job completion tasks are often done by
the High D **manager by**   antagonizing the team.
    Low D   avoiding the team.
    High I   conning people.
    Low I   distrusting the team members.
    High S   turning the crank harder.
    Low S   sacrificing his/her own health.
    High C   nit-picking.
    Low C   precipitating an argument.

Appendix D.4

People Compatibility by Behavior Characteristics

This chart is designed to give the user of the personality profile a few insights into compatibility of the different behavior types: D, dominant; I, inspirational; S, steady; and C, conscientious. Since most people have both highs and lows, at different intensities, on their charts, no single combination can be considered absolute. These are only indicators.

COMPATIBILITY ESTIMATE

Styles	Excellent		Good		Adequate		Poor	
	1	2	3	4	5	6	7	8
D-D				X	•			
D-I			X		•			
D-S		•				X		
D-C						•		X
I-I	X						•	
I-S	•				X			
I-C			•					X
S-S	X			•				
S-C		X		•				
C-C		X		•				

X = human (social) relations

• = work (task) relations

Appendix D.5

Procurement Information

Vendors

The D-I-S-C booklet is available from many sources, and the vendors listed below are not guaranteed or warranted by Catanzaro & Associates, Inc. We have found them to be competitively priced, so we offer them as an alternative to the original vendor:

- Padgett Thompson/Performax Systems International: 913-451-2700

- SourceCom: 800-433-3635+

- TAMCO: 800-657-2235

Available Resources (Prices May Change)

- *Personal Profile Manual* ($14.95). Useful tips on how to use the instrument for hiring, training, team building and counseling.

- *Personal Profile Audio Cassette.* A short cassette tape that talks the listener through the administration of the instrument.

- *Personal Profile System.* The instrument itself, sold in quantities. Prices as of fall 1998:

  D-I-S-C System booklets (2800) = $12.00 each
  D-I-S-C Overview booklet   = $4.50 each
  More than 25 System booklets   = $10.00 each

- *Personal Profile Package.* Three Personal Profile booklets, three worksheets, and one audio cassette.

- *Blueprint for Managing Differences.* Used with the Personal Profile System to assist in constructive interaction and dealing with conflict, both inside and outside the practice. You need to purchase the manual to get the full benefit from the Blueprint forms and exercise.

Staff Development Assessment

Managing a dynamic staff member can be one of the most challenging tasks a veterinary practice manager faces. The lack of in-service training often compounds even the most minor issues. This assessment can be used to assess the people skills of a practice manager candidate, as well as help you better understand the human resource alternatives available and how to manage around limitations. This assessment can also help you create the action plan (see Appendix F) when you initiate a change effort.

You will find 56 questions that will help you to assess your current understanding and knowledge of this management subject. You are asked to answer if you agree (A) or Disagree (DA) with any of the questions asked. If you are uncertain, choose the response that most closely matches your basic feeling about the question. Place an "X" in the box beside each statement that best describes how you feel. If you need to change your answer, simply draw a circle around the first "X," then mark a new "X" in the other box.

Issues	Agree	Disagree
1. Poor attitude staff members represent only 3 percent of a practice's team, but their costs equal 25 percent of payroll (in lost time, lower productivity, workman's comp, management time, medical costs).	❑	❑
2. At any one time, one-third to half of all supervisors report having problems with workers due to personal or emotional difficulties, lateness or absenteeism, or problems with work rules.	❑	❑
3. The weak staff member puts out about two-thirds the work of the average practice staff member.	❑	❑
4. Aetna states a problem employee has a 60 percent chance of more accidents than an average staff member.	❑	❑

Issues	Agree	Disagree
5. Problem staff members, as a group, are four times more likely to have alcohol or drug dependency problems than those staff members who perform acceptably.	❏	❏
6. Problem staff members have six times the lost time rate than the average nonproblem staff member.	❏	❏
7. Personality conflicts, personal problems, or poor attitudes contribute to most failures to meet outcome expectations.	❏	❏
8. According to surveys, the three hardest tasks for management are performance appraisal, employee discipline, and termination.	❏	❏
9. Half the time, staff members are brought to the administrator's attention because there has been a problem in training, or a middle manager has failed in his/her own function(s).	❏	❏
10. The best team-based practice areas should get new staff to train because winners make winners.	❏	❏
11. You can still maintain an excellent veterinary practice even with mediocre and poor attitude staff members.	❏	❏
12. Because management is reluctant or afraid, 50 percent of the problem staff members are not terminated.	❏	❏
13. Management training and development shouldn't be seen as an investment to control the costs of problem employees.	❏	❏
14. When excellent, well-trained managers deal with people correctly, formal disciplinary action becomes unnecessary.	❏	❏
15. It costs less to choose and hire good attitude staff members than to dehire (remove) unacceptable people from a practice team.	❏	❏

Issues	Agree	Disagree
16. If a practice doesn't properly orient new staff candidates, those new staff members could change the standards of the practice.	❑	❑
17. If staff members aren't used to the limit of their abilities, given bigger jobs, or stretched to do more, problems can be avoided.	❑	❑
18. When managers focus on disciplinary procedures and quasi-legal approaches, it creates animosity and distance between the staff and management.	❑	❑
19. When practices do not systematically reinforce or recognize good behavior, it can create negative staff reactions and confusion.	❑	❑
20. Positive job growth opportunities do not prevent problem behaviors from a few staff members.	❑	❑
21. Self-discipline is internal and voluntary and therefore most effective.	❑	❑
22. Sometimes counseling and other communication efforts are ineffective. If after two or three such attempts there is no positive response, chances are the person won't ever change and other courses of action should be attempted.	❑	❑
23. An authoritarian chewing out is less effective than a coaching or re-teaching approach.	❑	❑
24. Arranging consequences has proven more effective in changing behavior than trying to rely on communications for those cases in which problem attitudes/behaviors are deep seated.	❑	❑
25. The most successful counseling approach is to ask a series of questions, listen intently for answers, and guide the staff member to talk through problems.	❑	❑
26. Those staff members who overrate their own performances tend to be less than honest in reporting their shortcomings, and most are reluctant to make any changes in their behavior.	❑	❑

Issues	Agree	Disagree
27. Performance ratings tend to be mostly invalid, not usually legally defensible, and probably one of the biggest wastes of time.	❑	❑
28. Performance appraisals should be used primarily to plan individual development, determine goals, and set outcome objectives in practice performance.	❑	❑
29. Some managers tend to overreact and try to change some behaviors which aren't worth changing.	❑	❑
30. A staff member should be left uninformed of any file or documentation created regarding problem behaviors.	❑	❑
31. Positive as well as negative behaviors should be discussed during a staff member's counseling session.	❑	❑
32. Practice managers who deal with personnel tend to be too conservative and make it extremely difficult to fire poor performers.	❑	❑
33. Punishments are usually effective to turn people's problem attitudes around.	❑	❑
34. If any staff member's behavior is markedly improved over an agreed period of time, the past disciplinary record should be eliminated from the practice files.	❑	❑
35. Any staff member should be given three chances to improve before termination.	❑	❑
36. Managers should look for the most common signs of mental disturbance: extremes in personality, stress symptoms, out-of-control behavior.	❑	❑
37. Personal conduct problems are more difficult to correct than job performance problems.	❑	❑
38. Attendance cannot be improved by just defining the rules, applying penalties for absenteeism, keeping records of excessive absenteeism, or discussing reasons for absence.	❑	❑

Issues	Agree	Disagree
39. Those with alcohol abuse problems are more frequently absent on Mondays than on Fridays.	❏	❏
40. Threatened suspension or termination if a staff member doesn't change behavior works best for substance abusers.	❏	❏
41. Drug users tend to hold temporary jobs or lower skill jobs than they are capable of handling.	❏	❏
42. Accident-prone employees tend more to suffer from mental illness than the accident-free staff members.	❏	❏
43. Formal discipline rules are usually unnecessary since few veterinary staff members are truly disruptive.	❏	❏
44. Just so staff members don't make mistakes from ignorance, it's better to have lots of specific rules to cover many situations.	❏	❏
45. Any rule which is violated but not enforced is no longer a rule which can be enforced.	❏	❏
46. For formal discipline to work, a series of four warnings and an outside appeal process must be in effect.	❏	❏
47. A written and signed contract where appropriate behavior, review dates, conditions necessary for support, and standards for performance are spelled out is an effective approach to behavior control.	❏	❏
48. A more severe penalty can be imposed on those staff members with poor performance records.	❏	❏
49. Maintaining discipline is a negative function of management.	❏	❏
50. It is more humane and caring to keep poor performers in a job they can't do than to terminate them.	❏	❏

Issues	Agree	Disagree
51. A staff member should be fired to give him/her the chance to be successful somewhere else.	❏	❏
52. As soon as it's apparent a staff member hasn't responded to positive and negative disciplinary efforts, actions for termination should be initiated.	❏	❏
53. Any offense that requires suspension or termination should wait to be addressed until the end of the day or some other quiet time.	❏	❏
54. A veterinary practice is allowed by law, as a general principle, to terminate any staff member for any reason, good, bad, or indifferent, as long as (1) the reason is not specifically prohibited by law (e.g., discrimination) or (2) termination isn't directed at a contract employee.	❏	❏
55. Any decision to fire a staff member without documentation or evidence of step-by-step due process will be supported by any court of law.	❏	❏
56. In spite of any problems with a veterinary practice's case based on technicalities or deficiencies, the court will base its decision on three questions: (1) Was the employee fairly dealt with by the employer? (2) Was the process that led to termination objective? (3) Compared to other cases, is there evidence of consistency in this case?	❏	❏

STAFF DEVELOPMENT ASSESSMENT
Answers & Discussion

The following preferred answers and comments are a follow-up to each point in the situations contained in the Staff Development Assessment. They may not apply to your practice, but the discussion is always interesting when you ask, "How does this apply to our practice in the new millennium?" As you read through these comments, review carefully those answers you feel need attention in your veterinary practice; then look at the Action Plan in Appendix F for alternatives.

To Score this Questionnaire

While the scoring summary sheet is below, the actual preferred answer tally sheet is on the following page. The assessment is divided into eight sections; add the number of points in each section (based on preferred answers) and enter the scores in the appropriate score column under Raw Score. Then add up all the section scores to get the total. To help you see where your strengths are, rank order each of the sections. The highest rank equals 1, second highest 2, and so forth. If two sections scored equally, give them the same rank number. When done, bring your scores forward to the table below.

SCORING SUMMARY SHEET

Score Column	Raw Score	Rank
I. Problem Magnitude	_____	_____
II. The Manager's Role	_____	_____
III. Preventive Maintenance	_____	_____
IV. Counseling/ Performance Appraisal	_____	_____
V. Positive Corrective Actions	_____	_____
VI. The Exceptions	_____	_____
VII. Disciplinary Procedures	_____	_____
VIII. Termination	_____	_____
Total:	_____	_____

STAFF DEVELOPMENT ASSESSMENT
Answers and Tally Sheet

Problem Magnitude	Manager's Role	Preventive Maintenance	Counseling/ Performance Appraisal
1. A	8. A	15. A	22. A
2. A	9. A	16. A	23. DA
3. A	10. A	17. DA	24. A
4. A	11. DA	18. A	25. A
5. A	12. A	19. A	26. DA
6. A	13. DA	20. DA	27. A
7. A	14. DA	21. A	28. A
_____Subtotal	_____Subtotal	_____Subtotal	_____Subtotal

Positive Corrective Action	Exceptions	Disciplinary Procedures	Termination
29. A	36. A	43. A	50. DA
30. DA	37. A	44. DA	51. A
31. A	38. DA	45. DA	52. A
32. DA	39. DA	46. DA	53. DA
33. DA	40. A	47. A	54. A
34. A	41. A	48. DA	55. A
35. A	42. A	49. DA	56. A
_____Subtotal	_____Subtotal	_____Subtotal	_____Subtotal

Comments to the "Preferred Answers"

I. Problem Magnitude

1. **A.** Most veterinary practices try to kid themselves; these people are expensive. Either rehabilitate them or get them out.

2. **A.** These are the most frequent problems reported.

3. **A.** Part of this is caused by the time the staff member spends off the job, the other part by general performance problems.

4. **A.** Since these people tend to live out a sequence of problems, this can in-

clude safety violations. That's why it is important to take early corrective action rather than waiting for an accident to happen.

5. **A.** Careful here. Not all problem staff are alcoholics, and not all alcoholics are inept in performing their jobs or are being a problem. However, there is good probability that a problem staff member may be an alcoholic and that the poor behavior is a symptom of alcoholism.

6. **A.** Do not assume that a staff member only has an attendance problem. Lost time strongly indicates deeper problems are at work in the practice.

7. **A.** Incompetence and low job skills are only a small part of difficulties with problem staff members; the inattentive attitude toward patient care and other quality standards poses a major liability and is a forensic medical concern.

II. The Manager's Role

8. **A.** Note that the three hardest tasks fall under the category of problem staff members. Other hard tasks include work pressures and deadlines. See Chapter 6 of *Building the Successful Veterinary Practice: Programs & Procedures* (ISU Press) for alternatives to traditional performance appraisals that will spotlight the good staff members.

9. **A.** If you don't do your homework, you're bound to fail. Administrators must carefully select their people, set performance expectations, help the middle management train them to an acceptable trust level, communicate adequately, give praise for achievement, and do other positive things so their people aren't set up for failure. If the manager complains about a lot of problem people, chances are good the manager is the bigger problem.

10. **A.** Setting the level of expectation and ensuring the clarity of the outcome success measurement makes the difference between high performance, average performance, and low performance. Setting the example is the simplest way to get new team members tuned in to the level of performance truly desired.

11. **DA.** Don't bet your practice on it! Morale tends to drop, and new staff members may pick up on poor behaviors seen in the problem staff member who is getting away with murder. A single standard and clear expectations of performance, applied in an equitable and consistent manner, make staff harmony and practice quality an easier expectation.

12. **A.** No one said management was easy, and this task is certainly distasteful. Most practice owners have hired people in their own image and have seldom trusted their staff to be a hiring team. Some practice managers are uncertain how to proceed; therefore, they don't take action, and everyone suffers from the spread of the problem. We call the preferred separation process a dehiring, since everyone we hire has some good attributes; eventually, however, some staff evolve away from the practice direction or, in other cases, the practice evolves away from them. Sometimes this same inaction occurs when a new manager inherits the leftovers of past problems from his/her predecessor and is unsure which direction is acceptable to the practice.

13. **DA.** If you agreed with the statement, please pause to reflect. Those practice managers trained in handling people problems, staff or client driven, are better able to deal with the perceptions and feelings of others. These human resource trained managers feel more competent and confident doing so, and they usually get better results. Research shows that management development is one of the most cost-effective investments a veterinary practice can make and that it tends to reduce the costs caused by people problems.

14. **DA.** You can have a great practice administrator or hospital manager, but sometimes you have staff members who remain clueless. This is especially true when the practice owner or hospital director has delegated a closely held human resource program to a new administrator or manager. Many staff members will believe, "This too shall pass" and will just bide their time for the reversal of the delegation decisions. Disciplinary actions are a tool to provide an effective framework to deal with those people who haven't been smart enough to recognize the benefit of a good manager.

III. Preventive Maintenance

15. **A.** Do you realize most businesses still spend less time on selection than they do on correction? It's less expensive to train a manager in the art and science of interviewing, selection, and assessment procedures. There are, however, still those situations where you hire a good person who goes sour, or you unintentionally hire a person who was a problem the day they walked in the door. Train your managers. It takes more work, but it becomes less work and more pleasant than trying to rid yourself of problem people.

16. **A.** Since our work force has become more mobile and employment spans have shortened, it is vital that people learn the practice's expectations and culture. Those practices that don't manage this process find that the attitudes and beliefs of strangers have severely changed the atmosphere of their business and created internal situations that are impossible to manage. Spend the time in intensive orientation and avoid the cost of the rehabilitation of the candidate and the others affected.

17. **DA.** Don't underestimate your staff—**ever**. It's fine to start staff members at their approximate level of ability, but don't backwater them and condemn them to stagnation. The key to motivation is to stretch people, train to higher levels of competency, and push their capabilities to a higher level of performance.

18. **A.** When you're bogged down in policy, you lose sight of people and problems begin. Address people's needs for support first, then apply any necessary disciplinary tools. When you start to focus on appeals, grievances, writing up people, etc., the whole environment in the practice declines.

19. **A.** Why is it we received more gold stars and other warm fuzzies for recognized good performance when we were children, but the whole process becomes reversed in the traditional veterinary practice workplace? Parents, teachers, friends, coaches, and other important people in our lives usually set up conditioned expectations for recognition and praise for performance. Why should it stop just because we grew up and went to work? Why is it staff members only hear about what they've done wrong from doctors and managers, and then receive cold barbs of negative reinforcement, long after the fact, in the traditional appraisal process? The result is confusion, animosity, suspicion, paranoia, and other problems on the job.

20. **DA.** Look at the big picture. Want to prevent great frustration and buildups of steam that lead to problems? Consider career management devices and better job placement and human asset development. Most staff members will respond in a positive and harmonious way; the couple of old grouches out there probably work for someone else.

21. **A.** One definition of self-discipline is *the desire to perform well*. Managers can help put this definition into action through orientation and training, a positive work environment, good supervision, and all aspects of a healthy work environment.

IV. Counseling and Performance Appraisal

22. **A.** Counseling is not the answer to all problems. Emotionally disturbed staff members need referral to a professional. Good judgement dictates managers **not** spend too much time on a lost cause. If counseling doesn't work, try something else, such as a layoff or other consequence.

23. **DA.** Actually, it depends. Whatever communication style you use will depend on the personality with whom you're dealing and on what situation in the practice caused the conflicting behavior. It also depends on the current skill training situation and what the past communication with this person has been. When in doubt, start out nice—but then be more forceful if you aren't getting the person's attention. Since communication is a pragmatic art, use whatever works.

24. **A.** Behavior rewarded is behavior repeated. Actions speak louder than words (and continued counseling). Staff members have to know where the carrot is before they can chase it!

25. **A.** Here is where being designed with two eyes, two ears, and one mouth is a practical application of your natural physical attributes to the ratio the Lord gave you for communications. With questions and answers, you have the benefit of causative diagnostics as well as relationship interaction control. A second benefit is that you can help the staff member talk his/her way through to possible solutions to the problem. Then you have a better response from the staff member because it's his/her solution, not yours.

26. **DA.** How many people do you know who are that easy on themselves? About 90–95 percent of all staff members tend to rate themselves lower than their supervisor would rate them. Because of this, more practices have turned to self-evaluation as an approach to performance appraisal. The rating is still reviewed and discussed with the staff member by the supervisor/mentor, and the supervisor still has the final say. Of those 5–10 percent who rate themselves higher, one-half frequently do so innocently, but need to know where they are in their performance. The other 5 percent will be those who will always be difficult to counsel. However, most managers are highly satisfied with this approach because they've won with the other 95 percent without stress or an appraisal battle.

27. **A.** No matter what has been attempted, the process of performance rating usually is invalid and legally indefensible. It doesn't mean some approaches aren't better than others and worth doing (such as criterion-based, critical incident, peer review, self-evaluation). For the most part,

though, managers and staff agree; they indicate they get little or no value out of the process, which remains part of the old school of thought regarding subjective ratings.

28. **A.** Why dwell on the past other than to create a historical document or to build a case? People do need to know where they stand to prepare them to move to the next level of performance, as well as to see what work objectives are related to their responsibilities. We prefer the concept of *performance planning* (this sounds future tense) as a replacement terminology for *performance appraisals* (which sounds retrospective). Look forward with your people to help build them and the practice.

V. Positive Corrective Measures

29. **A.** Face it, people just have irritating, but harmless, behaviors. So don't waste your time letting them get to you, even if you are personally stressed and frustrated. Unless this behavior is unhygienic or detrimental to the practice or patients, and the bottom line, there's no need to bring it to the staff member's attention. Address issues, not personalities.

30. **DA.** There is no reason *not* to inform any staff member that a record has been created to serve as documentation. The styles of leadership start at directive training, then persuasion that they can do it, and eventually coaching while they are applying the skills and knowledge. Some documentation should be accolades, just as some may document recurring challenges in performance or behavior. The documentation is created by the supervisor to help communicate and control problems internally and, perhaps later, to be used in subsequent legal action. It also establishes the how seriously management takes the practice performance expectations. However, it isn't recommended that the staff member be allowed free access to the staff employee files (they should be treated as confidential files and kept secured).

31. **A.** However, beware of the proverbial *but*. Never offer a positive accolade with a *but* in the center of the statement. Accentuate the positive to help lead the staff member(s) away from the negative. This way, each person gets to feel the regard in which they are held and, therefore, will be more responsive to those specific areas of concern about their performance.

32. **DA.** Most veterinary practice managers tend to take the side of the staff, while many supervisors seem to be ready to share blame quickly. Often the doctors avoid any confrontation, forming a covert resistance to managers

who are having problems with a specific staff member. Taking the side of the staff member should only have to do with legal or policy requirements regarding how problems are to be handled (state or province wage and labor laws). Managers can get help from the practice owners to get problem people out of the practice, but it has to be done by the book.

33. **DA.** Maybe and maybe not. One has to look at the big picture of potential unpredictable behavior later on. Try a different approach first. If that works, the staff member doesn't carry around the negative feelings that result from punishment, and you both win.

34. **A.** People should be allowed to clear their records with no past misdeeds held over their heads. It does, however, make sense to insist on a long time period over which their behavior change remains stable. Otherwise, you may run into the problem of the staff member who behaves for six months, then falls back into old patterns. Clearing the record boils down to clear evidence of changed behavior rather than temporary compliance.

35. **A.** There are no hard and fast rules here, but if repeated offenses against expected job and personal standards are the norm for this person, there is a low probability of success for this person to be turned around. Forty chances is too many and often, one chance isn't enough. For the good of the practice, just don't let things linger too long.

VI. The Exceptions

36. **A.** These are the most common symptoms. The practice manager doesn't need to be able to label people or understand all the dynamics (administrators need to understand organizational behavior, but that is considered an advanced level of skills and knowledge). It is important, however, to recognize when people are more than upset and need professional assistance.

37. **A.** Job performance and expectations are a little more concrete than people's emotional states of mind. Many factors are at play in that arena. Therefore, to be more successful in handling a staff member's personal problems, the manager needs to know as much as possible about the person's background, personality, and motivation patterns. These considerations should not, however, delay or replace the person's possible need for professional counseling.

38. **DA.** An absentee surveillance program that utilizes these four factors stands a better chance of success. Unapproved absence, or tardiness, is

seen as a discourtesy to other staff members; in healthcare delivery, this cannot be tolerated. Most staff members test the system occasionally, and attendance is just one common area. Clear expectations, consistent consequences, documented behavior variances, and eye-to-eye remedial sessions with the leadership are critical in reestablishing the core values and mission focus of the practice.

39. **DA.** This is a common mistaken conception. Actual alcoholics' absences tend to be scattered throughout the work week, frequently as partial days of leaving early for some reason, rather than coming in late.

40. **A.** Anyone with a chemical dependency is disabled from responding to counseling or less severe consequences. The threat of job loss can be severe enough to drive him/her into counseling. Sometimes the supervisor's threat has been more successful in driving the person into rehabilitation than the spouse's attempts. In a healthcare setting, anything less puts patients in danger.

41. **A.** With skills impaired by drug use as well as a lower achievement drive caused by the drug, many users intentionally seek lower skill jobs that are beneath their capabilities. This way they can continue to function in a less demanding job and have the economic means to continue their habit.

42. **A.** Although not all accident victims are psychologically disturbed, a majority are. People with job accident histories are likely to repeat. As a form of self-punishment, this behavior allows them to survive off the practice (employer) without having to work. This behavior is termed a form of mental illness by experts in the field.

VII. Disciplinary Procedures

43. **A.** Although this is a true statement, even the occasional wayward staff member will justify the written policy. The policy sets the boundaries for all, especially for those who need to be fenced in.

44. **DA.** There is no need to write a policy manual like the Merck veterinary manual. No one can remember all that information without a photographic memory, so you have defeated your purpose. Enforced rules based on inviolate core values are more easily remembered than a lot of written rules that become lost in the brain or ignored.

45. **DA.** Just because a rule hasn't needed to be enforced doesn't mean it isn't enforceable. However, if it isn't enforced when the situation requires it, it might as well not exist. In cases where a rule is to be reinstated after long

disuse, management should inform the staff of the reenactment of the rule and that it will be used in the future.

46. **DA.** Don't tie up your practice with disciplinary bureaucracy. Keep it simple as you allow for a step-wise, due process review. Severe cases require no prior warnings other than at the initial orientation of a candidate for employment. In every case, however, enforcement of this discipline must be compatible with whatever approach the practice management uses.

47. **A.** Take the mystery out of expectations. Once signed, the contract makes clear that communication took place between the practice leadership and staff member and that the individual staff member agreed to the conditions set forth. Waffling doctor support behavior is greatly reduced by written contracts.

48. **DA.** The punishment should match the specific offense, not cumulative behavior which could unduly influence the penalty given. However, if the practice policy specifically allows for a cumulative approach to discipline, which then allows for a harsher penalty, the staff members need to know this up front, and the harsher penalty is then allowable.

49. **DA.** Who wants to manage anarchy? Remember, the word *discipline* comes from the Latin word *disciplina,* which means "teaching." As a more positive approach in management, discipline encompasses training, communication and counseling, and teaching by example. Harsher approaches are sometimes required, yet the outcome is still positive: to help people successfully correct their standards of performance.

VIII. Termination

50. **DA.** To be realistic would be more humane and caring; dehiring is essential when the practice and person have parted paths. Can you believe some managers actually use this thinking to justify not facing the difficulty of terminating someone? Don't they realize they are perpetuating a situation that keeps that person a terminal loser? Such thinking is also destructive to the individual's family life and his/her sense of self-esteem and self-respect; it also prevents the person from moving on to a better life elsewhere.

51. **A.** Sometimes you have to be cruel to be kind. Firing (we often call it dehiring to keep it in proper perspective), though most unpleasant, causes people to reevaluate what they are doing with their lives and allows them to move onward and upward. Evidence shows most people gain from this process. It's been reported by 80 percent of those terminated that after one

year they can claim, "It was the best thing that could have happened to me."

52. **A.** When you've exhausted all resources and alternatives, what choice is there? Do not delay separating those people who do not enjoy doing quality work or relating to the other members of the veterinary healthcare delivery team. To delay will drain group morale, create tension, and erode your practice standards.

53. **DA.** Why allow the poor performer time to stir up other staff members or commit some act of retribution. Those who know they are to be disciplined usually know it's coming. So move immediately.

54. **A.** This is known as *employment at will*. The major exceptions are employment contracts and such criteria as are specified by law (discrimination cases). Even though many feel the doctrine has been eroded in courts which are concerned about unjust firings and other badly handled approaches by employers, employment at will still means employers have the right to expect employees to meet standards of performance and conduct. They can remove employees who don't meet stated performance expectations. (Don't you just love this legal jargon?)

55. **A.** Believe it, especially if the violation is severe, such as stealing, causing physical harm, or exhibiting gross insubordination. The court might uphold employment at will without any documentation or due process; they may also uphold it for less severe violations, providing evidence of due process has been exhibited by the practice leadership.

56. **A.** There is seldom a perfect case in court. Both sides of the case will have defects in their arguments. However, the courts usually look for evidence of fairness, objectivity, and consistency on the employer's part. When considering how firm the ground is when dealing with a particular case, consider if those three variables are present.

Questions

How did your leadership team discussions go? How many times did you ask, how does this apply to our practice? Did you look at the lack of management job redesign or clear expectations as part of the problem, or were these part of the solution? How can you use these problem behavior situations to set a positive tone within your leadership expectations for practice performance? Are you ready?

Administrative Action Plans

How to Use these Action Plans

Staff development (see Appendix E) and *change management* (see Ready for Change Assessment in Chapter Five) are the two most confusing issues for most veterinary practices, and therefore, for practice managers, hospital administrators and, therefore, practice owners. These are true leadership issues, and they get more complex as the practice evolves from one level of operational format to another. These two documents will help you to think through various actions you might take to handle a specific emerging challenge, and in some cases when you are asleep at the wheel, add a step-by-step process for getting out of the rut you find yourself in without notice.

- For **each** challenge you work on, be sure to complete the appropriate action plan steps, and complete them in sequence whenever possible.

- When addressing a change using the sequence of the action plan, one discovery is often, "Oops, we forgot this step." In other cases, following the plan sequence prevents the quantum leap to an end point that may be a knee-jerk reaction (and thus detrimental to practice harmony and team success).

- To have an idea of what you've done up to this point, place a mark in the **Done** column next to those items on which you've already taken action.

- In most cases, practices become dysfunctional because what worked in a previous experience does not work in the current situation. It is not a bad practice, it is just a practice without adequate experience to know which paths of resolution are safe to tread upon (fear of failure is a given in healthcare professionals).

When you're finished with the preliminary list, go back through the list of suggested actions. In the **Need to Do** column, mark those items that need to be done. Later, when the tasks are completed, you can place a mark in the **Done** column. Finally, determine what needs to be done to create a calendar of events to coincide with these actions.

STAFF DEVELOPMENT ACTION PLAN

Step One: Introductory Case Assessment

Need to Do	Done	
❑	❑	1. Describe the person's problem. Include specifics and behavior. What should they start or stop doing?
❑	❑	2. Gather information to support and verify specific problems and their range.
❑	❑	3. Calculate what the problem person's behavior costs the team and how it impacts the practice.
❑	❑	4. Have a fact-finding discussion with the problem person to get his/her side of things.
❑	❑	5. Decide if this is a problem person or a person with a problem.

Step Two: Orientation and Training

Need to Do	Done	
❑	❑	1. Decide if the staff member is appropriate for the job. If not, consider a new role, redesigning the job, or dehiring (later steps).
❑	❑	2. Does person need recycling through orientation or job training? If this is basically an attitude or personality problem, don't rely on person's education to make a difference.
❑	❑	3. If the person is appropriate for the job but hasn't used the job skills lately, consider using more practice on the job. Consider a buddy system for this process.
❑	❑	4. If the job has changed, provide training in new skills.

Need to Do	Done	
❏	❏	5. Other observations: _____
		_____
		_____
		_____

Step Three: Counseling and Communications

Need to Do	Done	
❏	❏	1. Record factual information and any previous steps taken. Avoid including unsupported statements or opinions. Review historical staff documents to see if there is support for the current situation.
❏	❏	2. Decide if you want to help save the person or remove him/her from the practice. Are you personally close enough to the person to be able to help?
❏	❏	3. Schedule an informal, verbal, caring feedback session to review the facts, express your unhappiness with the recent behavior or attitude, and end with a positive belief that the person will correct his/her behavior or attitude.
❏	❏	4. Time to conduct a formal coaching session with the person. Be certain and clear of what the goals and objectives of the practice are, what behavior is expected, and what time factors are in effect.
❏	❏	5. Develop a written and signed performance contract with the staff member. Include objectives, applicable action plans, standards of performance, and dates for review and completion. Be sure these are realistic, measurable, and attainable.
❏	❏	6. Is there a personality conflict between you and the person which prevents successful turnaround of behavior or attitude? Consider referral actions (Step Four), but only if you believe there will be improved behavior and attitude with a new mentor.

Need to Do	Done	
❏	❏	7. You may need to use power counseling or the shape-up-or-ship-out talk. This approach requires you to have high self-confidence and a belief that the person is salvageable. This technique often includes the final written warning; review the dehiring procedures (Step Eight) so you'll be prepared in case the staff member is still unresponsive.
❏	❏	8. Other observations: _____

Step Four: Referral Actions

Need to Do	Done	
❏	❏	1. Stop further coaching and counseling efforts. You can take more direct action to refer the person if (a) two sessions have made little or no change in the person who seems upset or emotionally troubled or (b) three or four sessions have produced no results with an emotionally stable staff member.
❏	❏	2. You may need to refer the person to the leadership team for further action.
❏	❏	3. It may be time to refer the person to professional help.
❏	❏	4. You may need to refer the person to a consultant for further action.
❏	❏	5. Other observations: _____

Step Five: Managing the Reward System

Need to Do	Done	
❏	❏	1. If there are any organizational or environmental obstacles to the staff member's performance, remove them. These could be lack of resources, management support, time, etc.

Need to Do	Done	
❏	❏	2. If there are any existing penalties that prevent positive behavior, remove them. These could be poor practice norms or a new salary that is less than what was previously paid plus overtime.
❏	❏	3. Do not reward any type of poor behavior, such as pay for lost time or recognizing a person only when he/she misbehaves.
❏	❏	4. Develop new methods to reward positive behavior.
❏	❏	5. If any staff member demonstrates continued poor behavior or attitude, reduce the salary, cut any performance bonuses, reduce the job hours, or suspend them (with or without pay).
❏	❏	6. Other observations: _____

Step Six: Designing and Restructuring the Job

Need to Do	Done	
❏	❏	1. You may need to redesign the staff member's job to match his/her capabilities. If this isn't an option, is she/he capable of doing a different job?
❏	❏	2. Transfer the person to another shift, but only if you know that the problem won't be passing along to a new work team and that there will be improvement in the staff member's behavior.
❏	❏	3. Demote the person within his/her team, but only if this action is based on an in-practice job realignment procedure. It is often appropriate even when competence and good attitude are present.
❏	❏	4. Other observations: _____

Step Seven: Correctional Procedures

Need to Do	Done	
❏	❏	1. Use the practice's disciplinary or warning system. Follow the practice policy manual to communicate what is expected, what is wrong with the current performance, how the person could and should improve, when these improvements are expected, and the consequences if the staff member fails to act.
❏	❏	2. If you follow a step system, issue all appropriate verbal or written follow-up warnings.
❏	❏	3. Be sure to allow the staff member sufficient time, means, and support to improve.
❏	❏	4. Place the person on probation for a set period of time. If this doesn't work, you will be forced to de-hire the person.
❏	❏	5. Suspend the staff member with pay to give the leadership or management team time to review the case history and facts, and to allow the person time to see what else is available in the community. Suspension without pay is usually a form of punishment.
❏	❏	6. Any gross acts of misconduct, either by commission or omission, should never receive any step-wise progression. These are grounds for dismissal for cause.
❏	❏	7. Other observations: _____

_____

_____

_____

Step Eight: Termination Procedures

Need to Do	Done	
❏	❏	1. Review the entire situation with the leadership team or practice manager, whichever is most appropriate. This review may not lead to dehiring, but it certainly can help a manager who feels he/she did everything he/she could and needs a sort-it-out session.
❏	❏	2. Issue a final warning to the staff member, even though this isn't necessary in all cases.
❏	❏	3. Decide if the circumstances suggest support from outplacement services, such as job placement assistance, or more than the minimum severance pay or allowances.
❏	❏	4. Offer the staff member an opportunity to resign.
❏	❏	5. Dehire the staff member (job outgrew the person).
❏	❏	6. Prepare for anxiety or celebration from the rest of the practice team. Will there be any need for damage control?
❏	❏	7. Review what went wrong to avoid this problem in the future.
❏	❏	8. Other observations: _____

Summary of Needed Actions

After you've selected your **Need to Do** action items, enter them in the following grid in the sequence that makes the most sense for you to deal with the situation.

Action number	Specific action needed	Operational notes (mentor, etc.)	Date to begin	Date to be completed

Note: If you need any help or further ideas regarding this Staff Development Action Plan, feel free to contact Veterinary Practice Consultants®, Catanzaro & Associates, Inc., at 303-277-9800, fax 303-277-9888, or e-mail Cat9800@ aol.com.

CHANGE ASSESSMENT ACTION PLAN

This document will help you to think through various aspects of managing a change you intend to make in your practice. The models and sequences in this action plan will make you assess if you have covered all relevant matters. Use only those sections and exercises that are appropriate to your efforts toward change.

I. How to Manage the Change Formula

You need to determine if your proposed change will measure up to the following formula:

$$C = D \times M \times P > Costs$$

If it doesn't, you could be in serious trouble, or worse, fail.

The Formula Defined

C = Change. The best change only occurs when each of the other factors (**D, M,** and **P**) are present in equitable quantity. If any of these factors are absent or small in quantity, your practice change effort will not occur as a smooth process. Also, interaction among **D, M,** and **P** needs to be positive enough that the benefits of any change will outweigh the costs of the change.

D = Dissatisfaction/Desire. When conditions are uncomfortable, change most often occurs, but not usually because of positive desire. **D** represents the pressure to change through internal factors, such as doctor or staff unhappiness, or through external forces, such as competition or government regulations. **D** also is the energy required for change to occur and frequently can be the result of a crisis or of relevant, accurate, and supported data. The practice manager's role is to increase the desire (**D**) to energize the organization need for change.

M = Model. **M** is the leader's vision for new, positive methods to do things, think, feel, and behave (it must have crystal clear clarity and fit the practice vision). To create a lot of **D** without **M** results in blame and finger pointing. People don't know what to do. Many traditional veterinary managers can provide **M**, the picture of what should be, but often cannot provide **P**.

P = Participative Process. P provides the means for individuals or teams affected by change to work through their resistance and reach a point of acceptance. The process includes communication, participation, and time. Mistakes are usually made in top-down or bottom-up processing where the higher or lower levels of the organization try to influence each other. Wherever time allows, the best approach is a cyclical **P** where different levels in the practice staff assess the benefits of the **M**, then look for reactions from others who are affected. Such involvement usually leads to acceptance.

The following exercise assesses whether you have adequately provided for all the necessary factors involved so that positive change can occur. **Always** ask yourself and your leadership team, "Which of the following factors need more work in our practice?"

A. Creating Dissatisfaction/Desire

1. Other than yourself, who will provide the energy for change? Who is dissatisfied with the current situation, or who wants it better? How can one personally use one's own energy source to increase **D**? What/who is going to push through the change? A common failure in change is underestimating the amount of physical, emotional, and intellectual energy required. Do you and the others have the staying power needed?

---

2. How can the **D** be communicated or spread throughout the practice in a positive manner? How could **D** be increased creatively (for example, build on strengths)? What examples or information could be used to spread **D** and gain supporters for change?

B. Developing an Adequate Model

1. What is the **M** needed in your practice's future? What precise model, plan, or picture needs to be developed that specifies the outcome expectations (such as a new program-based budgeting process)? What ways can this modeling be clarified/simplified/visualized? What improvements to the outcome accountability model need to be clarified (such as success measurements)?

_____

_____

_____

2. What are two ways to break down the model into stages (a small-bite time line) to make communication, acceptance, or implementation easier (such as staff selects from two yes alternatives)?

_____

_____

_____

3. Can you test a pilot model for 90 days instead of jumping into the unknown? Who would defend this pilot test from those who are against it?

_____

_____

_____

C. Obtaining Acceptance from Those Affected

1. **P** is the term used to describe how people finally reach the point of accepting their participation in the process. Can others be persuaded to embrace the change? How can the change be made relevant to their specific interests? Can elements be negotiated, rather than compromised, to create leverage for others to want to support the change?

_____

_____

_____

2. Are there any rewards or recognitions that could be used to support the pursuit of change? How can rewards be withdrawn from those who resist change? What's in it for those affected? Would it be a good idea to analyze people's positions to determine what forces affect them? Is there any glory which could be shared?

_____

_____

_____

3. Can those who are affected help to shape the model? Can they design, test, and train it before it is fully implemented? Does their staff position in the practice affect this question?

_____

_____

_____

4. Is it possible to make the change fun, enjoyable, and positive? Can any sub-goals or early results be celebrated? How can satisfaction of achievement be made real and available to the participants? Since celebration is essential to change, how can it be sustained?

_____

_____

_____

D. Benefit/Cost Ratio

Remember: change usually occurs only if the benefits of **D × M × P** are greater than the costs. First, you need to identify the benefits and costs of the change you're contemplating. Benefits to the clients or staff in the practice could be in economic areas, operating efficiency, service, personal/professional advancement, practice liquidity, or competitive advantage. Costs might be expense, time and effort, organizational paralysis, threats to personal status, job security, or competency. Next, you want to assign a point value from 1 to 10 for each element (1 = low, 10 = high). Total your figures to see if the benefits outweigh the costs by a substantial margin.

Change Areas	Benefit Points	Cost Points
Client-centered	_____	_____
Patient advocacy	_____	_____
Staff harmony	_____	_____
Liquidity	_____	_____
Practice image	_____	_____
Total:	_____	_____

II. Measure the Environment and Change the Situation

A. History

Can you identify anything that happened in, around, or about the practice culture where you operate that could affect your planned change? What happened in the past that could impact the present (such as changes in management direction, competition, regulations, economics, morale, reporting relationships, new products, consultant reports, etc.)?

Recent or Historical Factor or Event	Impact or Influence on Planned Change
_____	_____
_____	_____
_____	_____
_____	_____

B. Strategic Response Analysis

Change always is available from what we call *a strategic assessment.* Certain community and practice issues become driving forces, requiring change, while other limitations restrain them. First identify these factors; then develop a strategic response to deal with them.

Driving Forces

Driving forces favor your change and may include such things as the practice culture, potential for profit, benefits and rewards, popularity of the change, and the key power people. Identify all the driving forces currently operating in your situation. Consider any other force factors which could be added to this list. How can each of these forces be strengthened or their potential increased?

Driving Forces	Strengthen By
_____	_____
_____	_____
_____	_____
_____	_____
_____	_____
_____	_____

Restraining Forces

Restraining forces resist change. They may include cost, lack of time, human insecurities, regulations/policies/precedents, opposition or relationships among key players, or simple inertia. Identify all the restraining forces. Can any of them be removed from the list or at least neutralized? Of those that remain, how can their influence be lessened or moderated?

Restraining Forces	Weaken or Deal With By
_____	_____
_____	_____
_____	_____
_____	_____
_____	_____
_____	_____

C. Does It Fit?

The following steps will help you think through whether it's possible to make the change you're considering so you don't charge ahead into the unknown. There are three tests. A failure in one could represent a failure for your planned change.

Test 1

Is there a reasonable fit between the size of the change contemplated and your power within the practice? If not, is the change too big to even attempt? Can it be reduced to a workable size?

_____

_____

Test 2

Is there a reasonable fit between the end result of what is to be done and the practice's realities/imperatives that make up the culture of the current environment? In other words, what is possible with this client base in terms of the change itself? If nothing can be done, can the model for the end result be changed?

_____

_____

Test 3

Is there a reasonable fit between the readiness of key individuals and the practice team for change (their attitudes, skills, and dissatisfaction energy and the change method you intend to use)? The change method usually will be either a participative approach where you work on attitudes first, then make the change, or a very directive approach where you make the change first, then work on people's attitudes.

_____

_____

III. DEALING WITH RESISTANCE

It is normal to resist change. It is expected. In healthcare delivery, stasis of any system or entity means death, but when we are operating a veterinary practice, the desire is for replication of the successful procedures, consistency, and continuity of care. Many administrators and managers confuse the healthcare delivery needs with the practice business needs; business operations do not seek stasis—ever! While the participative method of developing the process you've planned will help reduce the resistance, it's good to be prepared for some problems arising. Which of the following resistance factors will be part of your change situation?

A. Why People Balk at Change

- Lack of understanding or poor communication.
  - ✓ Fear the unknown.
  - ✓ Not understanding the change or seeing the need for it.
  - ✓ Lack of communication about the change or getting the news secondhand.
  - ✓ Inability to prepare, not knowing how to perform.

- Losses or costs of change.
  - ✓ Perceived job loss.
  - ✓ Comfort with the present way things are done.
  - ✓ Feeling that the change won't be beneficial.
  - ✓ Cost is too great in terms of personal life, competence, confidence, and relationships.
  - ✓ Any self-investment and creativity put into current method, any perceived disposal of present system considered a rejection of "my baby."

- No participation or control.
  - ✓ Fear of not fitting into the group norms or that change acceptance will lead to social isolation from peers.
  - ✓ Not asked for any input regarding the change—a feeling of being cogs in the machine, leading to minimal compliance.
  - ✓ Unable to shape or alter the change, which leads to passive resistance as a way to hide true feelings.

- Attitudinal problems or emotional reactions.
  - ✓ Negative mind set about the job or practice to begin with, expressed by resistance.
  - ✓ Change taken as personal criticism and a slap in the face of one's competence.
  - ✓ Dislike of the person who introduces change due to long-time bad relationship.
  - ✓ Immature attitude which creates a "bad attitude."
  - ✓ Defensive reactions to protect their status quo comfort, such as rationalizing, delaying, or placing blame onto someone else.
  - ✓ Less personal commitment to the practice than what process or model expects.

- Legitimate work concerns.
  - ✓ Timing is bad, too much work to do for individuals and practice.
  - ✓ Insufficient resources or other causes perceived to cause change to fail.
  - ✓ Change is seen as unethical, incorrect, or a violation of values.
  - ✓ Expected to change with no direction given as to how or what to do.
  - ✓ Sees the change as too complex, ambiguous, or without an adequate implementation plan.

B. Planning for Those Who Balk

In most practices, the doctors and administrators need to prepare in advance for the above resistance factors. The hospital administrator or practice manager(s) and owners must have a common approach to conflict resolution, and the practice management structure needs a full internal support plan, so on any project or change action, consider an early meeting to fill in the following information:

Resistance Person/Group	Resistance Factors	How to Handle It

IV. Action Planning and Next Steps

The following items are key in leading to various change efforts. Use these experience-proven questions to test how adequate your preparation is. First check off those items that are **done** so you have a clear picture of where you are now. Then go back through the list and check those items you **need to do.**

A. Play into the Change Formula

Need to Do	Done	
❑	❑	Increase the Dissatisfaction with the present way of doing things among staff and associates.
❑	❑	Refine the Model to make it more simple, comprehensive, easier to understand, more appealing.
❑	❑	Improve the Process by:

		Need to Do	Done	
		❑	❑	Establishing a communication plan
		❑	❑	Talking with team leaders
		❑	❑	Talking with individual staff members

Need to Do	Done	
❏	❏	Talking with staff as a group in meetings
❏	❏	Assigning members of staff to certain parts of the project
❏	❏	Accepting workable staff input
❏	❏	Announcing any changes as far in advance as possible

Need to Do	Done	
❏	❏	Review the whole situation regarding both planning and implementation, assess team strengths, and change Dissatisfaction into Desire for change.

B. Controlling the Situation

Need to Do	Done	
❏	❏	Understand the history that has influenced this situation.
❏	❏	Reinforce the current practice vision and leadership climate in the plan.
❏	❏	Determine the timing and appropriateness of the change. Take into account the amount of past change the practice has undergone and the realities of the present situation.
❏	❏	Add to or strengthen your list of driving forces.
❏	❏	Shorten or weaken your list of restraining forces.
❏	❏	Add to your list of benefits. Look for additional values to support the change, such as rewards, status, responsibility, achievement, independence, working relationships, etc. Find the hot buttons of each key player.
❏	❏	Reduce your list of costs and their potential penalty size.
❏	❏	Combine an unpopular change with a popular change.
❏	❏	Earn the respect and acceptance as the change leader from the rest of the practice staff.
❏	❏	A test: will it be possible for you as the change leader to maintain the physical, intellectual, and emotional energy required?

C. Develop the Work Plan

Need to Do **Done**

❑ ❑ Estimate as correctly as you can the time and resources required to support the change effort. Remember that everything takes longer, is harder, and costs more than you think. Have you planned for additional time in case of delays? What about extra money for budget overruns?

❑ ❑ Determine risks both to yourself and the key supporters.

❑ ❑ Determine the practice's risks.

❑ ❑ Identify the basic commitments and determine what might need to be redesigned.

❑ ❑ Spell out the process, the model, and your time line.

❑ ❑ Share outcome expectations and use joint planning rather than the rumor mill to help others deal with their worry work.

❑ ❑ Be decisive on small, common sense issues to set the tone.

❑ ❑ Prepare yourself for more work than what was anticipated.

D. Political Savvy (especially critical for contract administrators)

Need to Do **Done**

❑ ❑ Find staff supporters for the change effort.

❑ ❑ Decide if your timing is right.

❑ ❑ Decide if you can aggressively pursue the total change or if you must do it in small increments.

❑ ❑ Listen carefully to your supporters in the practice.

❑ ❑ A test: are you being realistic? Or have you grabbed a tiger by the tail?

❑ ❑ Be sure to support other people's personal agendas along with your planning of the project.

❑ ❑ Be sure to balance a staff member's interests with some of the staff member's perceived bargaining positions.

❑ ❑ Make that road to change as smooth as possible for everyone.

Need to Do	Done	
❏	❏	Remember that your change management emphasizes the participation process more than the model building. The model *will* change in most all practice situations.
❏	❏	Remember that to master change, people need doctor and leader support, and that must be client centered or staff centered, not just task oriented.

Note: If you need any help or further ideas regarding this Change Assessment Action Plan, or if you need a change agent's assessment of your needs, please contact Veterinary Practice Consultants®, Catanzaro & Associates, Inc., at (303)277-9800, fax (303)277-9888, or e-mail Cat9800@aol.com.